A Patient's Guide to Clinical Trials

A Patient's Guide to Clinical Trials

Navigating the Promise and Pitfalls of Experimental Treatments

Jose-Alberto Palma, MD, PhD

BLOOMSBURY ACADEMIC
NEW YORK • LONDON • OXFORD • NEW DELHI • SYDNEY

BLOOMSBURY ACADEMIC
Bloomsbury Publishing Inc, 1359 Broadway, New York, NY 10018, USA
Bloomsbury Publishing Plc, 50 Bedford Square, London, WC1B 3DP, UK
Bloomsbury Publishing Ireland, 29 Earlsfort Terrace, Dublin 2, D02 AY28, Ireland

BLOOMSBURY, BLOOMSBURY ACADEMIC and the Diana logo
are trademarks of Bloomsbury Publishing Plc

First published in the United States of America 2026

Copyright © Jose-Alberto Palma, 2026

Cover design: Jen Huppert
Cover image © Getty/Vicki Jauron, Babylon and Beyond Photography

All rights reserved. No part of this publication may be: i) reproduced or transmitted in any form, electronic or mechanical, including photocopying, recording or by means of any information storage or retrieval system without prior permission in writing from the publishers; or ii) used or reproduced in any way for the training, development or operation of artificial intelligence (AI) technologies, including generative AI technologies. The rights holders expressly reserve this publication from the text and data mining exception as per Article 4(3) of the Digital Single Market Directive (EU) 2019/790.

Bloomsbury Publishing Inc does not have any control over, or responsibility for, any third-party websites referred to or in this book. All internet addresses given in this book were correct at the time of going to press. The author and publisher regret any inconvenience caused if addresses have changed or sites have ceased to exist, but can accept no responsibility for any such changes.

A catalog record for this book is available from the Library of Congress.

ISBN: HB: 979-8-8818-4247-5
ePDF: 979-8-2163-5203-7
eBook: 979-8-2163-5169-6

Typeset by Integra Software Services Pvt. Ltd.
Printed and bound in the United States of America

For product safety related questions contact productsafety@bloomsbury.com.

To find out more about our authors and books visit www.bloomsbury.com and sign up for our newsletters.

To my wife, for her endless patience and love.
For all the patients who teach us more than we teach them.
To my children, who remind me what matters.

Contents

Why I Wrote This Book x

Introduction 1
    How to Use This Book 4

1 Understanding Clinical Trials: A Primer 7
    What Is a Clinical Trial? 7
    Overview of the Clinical Trial Phases 16
    Must All Drugs Complete Every Phase? 22
    Overview of the Drug Development Process 25
    Who Is Responsible and Pays for a Clinical Trial? 28
    Who Oversees Clinical Trials? 29
    Ten Clinical Trials Myths 32
    Chapter 1 Highlights 35

2 Should You Join a Clinical Trial? 37
    The Good, the Bad, and the Ugly: Real-World Cases of Extreme Success or Failure 38
    Why People Participate in Clinical Trials 42
    Understanding Potential Clinical Trial Risks and Burdens 46
    Placebo, Blinding, Randomization, and Other Uncertainties 50
    The Three Most Important Questions to Ask Yourself 57
    How to Discuss Clinical Trials with Your Doctor 58
    Chapter 2 Highlights 62

3 Where to Start: Finding Clinical Trials 65
    How to Search for Clinical Trials 66
    A Step-by-Step Guide to Using ClinicalTrials.gov 70

Can Artificial Intelligence Chatbots Help to Find
Clinical Trials? 77
Other Resources and Websites for Finding Trials 79
When No Trials Are Available 87
Is It a Clinical Trial or a Scam? 94
Chapter 3 Highlights 97

4 Choosing the Right Clinical Trial 99

Key Questions before Selecting a Trial 100
Ranking Clinical Trials: How to Prioritize Your Options 102
Learning More about the Experimental Therapy and
Its Target 112
Becoming a Participant in a Clinical Trial 117
What Happens If a Trial Is Delayed or Canceled? 122
Chapter 4 Highlights 126

5 Inside the Clinical Trial: What to Expect 129

The Informed Consent Is the First Step of the Screening 130
Understanding Trial Criteria and Confirming Eligibility 139
What Is a Screen Failure? 143
After the Screening: Randomization and Additional Visits 144
Participants' Responsibilities and Commitment 147
What Happens If You Want to Stop Your Participation in
a Trial? 153
Chapter 5 Highlights 155

6 Practical and Emotional Support during the Trial 157

Financial and Medical Insurance Implications 158
Travel and Logistics Planning 163
Balancing Work, Family, and Trial Commitments 167
How Caregivers Can Support Trial Participants 169
Building a Support Network 173
What to Do When Things Go Wrong 177
Chapter 6 Highlights 179

7 After the Trial: What Comes Next? 181

What Happens at the End-of-Study Visit? 182

Open-Label Extension 184
Pros and Cons of OLE Participation 188
What If an Open-Label Extension Is Not Available? 190
Do Clinical Trial Participants Feel Valued? 192
Accessing Clinical Trial Data and Results 193
Handling Negative Clinical Trial Results 197
Integrating Clinical Trial Results into Your Healthcare 199
Support Systems after the Trial 201
Chapter 7 Highlights 204

8 Addressing Unique Populations in Clinical Trials 207

Clinical Trials in Children 208
Clinical Trials in Other Vulnerable Populations 215
Clinical Trials for Rare Diseases 221
Increasing Representation in Clinical Trials 225
Chapter 8 Highlights 229

9 The Future of Clinical Trials: Innovation and Empowerment 231

How Could Drug Development and Clinical Trials Be Improved? 232
Decentralized Clinical Trials: Clinical Trials at (or Near) Home 237
AI and Digital Technologies 239
Could We Ever Get Rid of Clinical Trials? 245
The Most Important Innovation: Empowered Participants 247
Chapter 9 Highlights 249

Epilogue: Considering Clinical Trials—A Leap of Hope 251
Acknowledgments 254
Resources for Further Information 256
Glossary 265
Selected Bibliography 271
Index 273
About the Author 279

Why I Wrote This Book

Clinical trials have been at the center of my professional life for over fifteen years. I've designed them, conducted them, and, most importantly, walked patients and their families through the complex, often overwhelming journey of participating in them. But my connection to clinical trials isn't just professional; it's personal. And that's why I wrote this book.

My journey in clinical research began in academia. As a physician-scientist at the New York University (NYU) Grossman School of Medicine, a premier medical and academic institution, I had the privilege of leading neurodegeneration clinical trials, working closely with thousands of patients and caregivers. I saw firsthand the hope these studies could bring and the frustrations, fears, and difficult decisions they often entailed.

Often, patients would sit across from me, grappling with uncertainty, and time and again, they would ask the same question: "Doctor, do you have a book or guide that I can read to learn more about clinical trials?"

It was a fair question. There are countless technical and scientific books on clinical trial design and statistical analysis, but nothing I could confidently hand to a patient, nothing that explained the process in clear, accessible terms while addressing both the medical and emotional realities of trial participation.

After a decade of academic work, I transitioned to the pharmaceutical industry to take on a global leadership role in neurodegeneration trials, first at Novartis and then at Eli Lilly, while still maintaining a part-time appointment at NYU. On this side of the table, my mission remained the same: to help patients by developing novel treatments. I focused on designing clinical trials that were scientifically rigorous and as patient friendly as possible, collaborating with academic physicians and advocacy groups to ensure that trials were accessible, ethical, and truly meaningful.

Then, shortly after the COVID-19 pandemic, clinical trials became personal. My mother was diagnosed with a rare, aggressive cancer that advanced far too quickly. Despite all my expertise, I found myself in the same position as so many patients and families I had counseled: scrambling for options, deciphering eligibility criteria, and trying to navigate a system that often feels cold and impenetrable. We tried to move fast, but the disease moved faster. My mother passed away before she could enroll in a trial. That experience changed me. It drove home just how overwhelming and exhausting this process can be, even for those with medical training, and how desperately patients and caregivers need clear, compassionate guidance when every moment counts.

This book is that guide. It's the resource I wish had existed when I was searching for options for my mother, and the resource I'd want others to have now. It's the knowledge I've shared with patients, families, friends, and colleagues throughout my career, now in a format that's accessible to anyone facing the daunting world of clinical trials.

My goal is simple: to empower you with the knowledge you need to make informed decisions, advocate for yourself or your loved one, and approach the process with confidence. Clinical trials aren't just about science or medicine; they're about people—people seeking a chance at something better.

If this book can make even one person's journey a little bit easier, then it has served its purpose.

Introduction

Receiving a diagnosis of an incurable disease, perhaps an unfamiliar condition you never imagined facing, can feel like your world has been turned upside down. Shock, fear, disbelief, and uncertainty are natural reactions. This news may carry an added burden for caregivers, amplifying the sense of helplessness while deepening the determination to provide support. As the doctor delivered the devastating news, you might have been desperate for answers and guidance. The only hope, the doctor tells you, the only chance to improve your odds of survival could be a clinical trial drug.

But what clinical trial? How can you find it? How can you ensure that you're eligible and can access the drug? Studies[1] highlight that nearly half of people know *nothing at all* about clinical trials, and around 60 percent would turn to their healthcare provider for more information. This seems reasonable, right? The problem is that while many doctors are skilled at diagnosing diseases, most are not familiar with the intricacies of clinical trials. Consequently, healthcare providers usually provide incomplete answers, leaving patients and caregivers stranded in a maze with no map or direction. Most healthcare providers not involved in clinical trial research may offer imprecise advice, like "Just check the website of this or that hospital (usually Mayo Clinic or Memorial Sloan Kettering Cancer in New

York City)—they do a lot of trials." This might be useful if you are lucky, and these hospitals have an open clinical trial that matches your diagnosis and stage of the disease. But what if they don't have any trial that fits you?

Despite the potential benefits of clinical trial participation, only a fraction of eligible patients (just 8 percent of adults with cancer,[2] for example) ever participate in trials.

Why don't more patients participate in trials?

One major barrier is the lack of clear, accessible information. Many patients don't know how to find clinical trials or fully understand their purpose, risks, and potential benefits. This information gap prevents thousands from exploring what might be lifesaving options. On top of that, the clinical trial process itself is complex, often overwhelming, not just for patients and families but even for many healthcare providers. Simply put, the clinical trials world is not designed with patients in mind.

This book recognizes these challenges and aims to empower all readers with the knowledge and resources to make informed decisions about clinical trials. Whether you're starting to think about trials, actively searching for a trial, evaluating its risks and benefits, or trying to understand what to expect after participation, this book provides the tools and insights you need to move forward with confidence.

You may want to take your best shot at prolonging your own life or the life of your loved one. Or perhaps you have a condition that isn't life threatening but still impacts your quality of life and you want to explore experimental treatments. This book will help you:

- find and evaluate available clinical trials;
- determine whether you might be eligible to participate;
- assess the risks and benefits of the trials;

- understand why placebos are often necessary;
- understand the differences among clinical trial phases;
- decide if a trial is the right choice for you (the answer might be no!); and
- identify potential economic costs and logistical challenges.

Importantly, the book also explains what happens after a trial ends, and explores the possibilities that may lie ahead.

Patients and caregivers are the primary audience for this book. You may not have a life-threatening disease and simply want to learn more about clinical trials, or perhaps you are a healthy volunteer considering participating in a trial to help advance science. That's perfectly fine; this book is for you, too. I also hope doctors and healthcare providers unfamiliar with the clinical trial process will find this book valuable to support their patients.

For those who have received a devastating diagnosis, access to clear information about clinical trials may be their only glimmer of hope. Sometimes, the hope is for a cure that can eradicate the disease. Other times, it's to alleviate symptoms, improve quality of life, or slow disease progression to gain more time. More time to spend with loved ones. More time to play with grandchildren. More time to resolve unfinished business or make plans. More time to cherish your memories. More time to forgive or seek forgiveness. Depending on the therapy and its success, the added time may be short. Sometimes just a few weeks. Still, for many, the quest to find that ray of hope is worth pursuing. If this is your case, I hope this book will make your journey easier.

As you embark on this challenging journey, know that you are not alone. This book is your companion, filled with practical advice, real-life stories, and clear guidance to help you navigate the complexities of clinical trials. With knowledge, courage, and hope, you can take confident steps toward making informed decisions for yourself or your loved ones.

How to Use This Book

The book has been organized into chapters, each including a summary of key points. Additionally, look for these helpful features throughout the book:

1. Definitions, denoted by a book symbol 📖, highlight key terminology, providing clear explanations of essential terms to ensure you have a solid understanding of the foundational ideas discussed throughout the book.
2. Caution, denoted by a warning symbol ⚠, brings attention to important concepts to help you avoid misunderstandings or poor decisions.
3. Case in Point, denoted by a magnifying glass symbol 🔍, provides real-life examples or personal stories that bring key concepts to life. To protect privacy, some personal details, such as names, may have changed.
4. Pro Tips, denoted by a light bulb symbol 💡, offer practical advice to simplify your journey and enhance your experience.

Depending on your situation, you may find it helpful to start with a specific chapter. If you're urgently searching for a clinical trial, begin with Chapter 3, which explains how to familiarize yourself with search tools, and outlines strategies to find potential trials and assess your eligibility. If you already have a few trials in mind, skip ahead to Chapter 4 to learn how to evaluate your options and make an informed choice. If you're unsure whether participating in a clinical trial is the right decision, start with Chapter 2, which outlines the risks, benefits, and considerations involved. Caregivers looking for ways to support a loved one during a trial may find Chapter 6 especially helpful.

No matter where you begin, this book is designed to guide you through every stage of the clinical trial process.

Bolded words are explained in the glossary at the end of the book. If a bolded term is unfamiliar, consult the glossary for a clear definition.

Notes

1. The survey can be accessed at https://hints.cancer.gov/docs/Briefs/HINTS_Brief_48.pdf (March 25, 2025).

2. According to Judy Sewards, head of clinical trial experience at Pfizer, during a panel discussion on clinical trials during the "2023 STAT Future Summit": https://www.statnews.com/2023/09/07/cancer-clinical-trials-diversity/; other estimates are even lower; for instance, only 1.7 percent of patients with an incident (new) cancer diagnosis participated in clinical trials between 2000 and 2002, as published in Vivek H. Murthy, Harlan M. Krumholz, and Cary P. Gross, "Participation in Cancer Clinical Trials: Race-, Sex-, and Age-Based Disparities," *Journal of the American Medical Association* 291, no. 22 (June 2004): 2720–26.

1

Understanding Clinical Trials: A Primer

You've picked up this book because you're looking to learn how to find a clinical trial and decide if it's the right fit for you or your loved one. Before diving into that topic, though, we need to start with the basics: understanding what a clinical trial is, the typical phases involved, and how the **drug** development process works. While it might seem tedious, these definitions and classifications are crucial for understanding the role of clinical trials in drug development, and how to distinguish legitimate studies from fraudulent ones. Stick with me, and we'll navigate these essentials together.

What Is a Clinical Trial?

Clinical trials are one type of clinical research study, which investigate various aspects of health and illness in people. But not all research studies are clinical trials. To understand what clinical trials are, let's first look at what they aren't.

Imagine a study where researchers ask two groups of adults, one with Parkinson's disease and one without, about their past exposure to pesticides. They aren't testing a treatment (i.e., it is a noninterventional study) but gathering data to answer a question: Could pesticide exposure increase the risk of Parkinson's? While this is not a clinical trial, noninterventional studies like this help identify risk factors for diseases. Once researchers understand these risks, they can work on therapies to address them, therapies that could eventually be tested in clinical trials. In this example, identifying a specific pesticide that is linked to Parkinson's disease may open the door to understanding the action of this pesticide in the brain and trying to develop a potential therapy that reverses or prevents that poisonous action. Once researchers develop a therapy and confirm its safety in animals, it's time for the next big question: Will it work in humans? That's where clinical trials come in.

⚠ Knowing the difference between clinical trials and other research studies is crucial. Why? Because databases like ClinicalTrials.gov list both, and it's easy to confuse the two. For example, a study titled "Clinical Trial Readiness for Genetic Epilepsy" might sound like a clinical trial but isn't. It's a noninterventional study aimed at developing future trial tools like biomarkers or disease scales.

Table 1.1 Examples of Noninterventional Studies and Clinical Trials

Noninterventional Studies	Clinical Trials
Study links e-cigarette use to lung cancer risk	Test if a novel chemotherapy extends survival in lung cancer
Observe brain volume changes in Alzheimer's	Test if an antibody slows brain atrophy in Alzheimer's
Analyze gene mutation association with colon cancer	Test if a gene therapy can prevent colon cancer

📖 **Clinical trials** are clinical research studies that test the effect of an intervention on health-related biomedical or behavioral outcomes in humans.

Let's break down the definition into its four key concepts: "test," "intervention," "human," and "health-related biomedical or behavioral outcomes." Each plays a critical role in defining what makes a clinical trial unique.

Clinical Trials Are Tests

Clinical trials are research tests designed to answer key questions: Is the intervention safe? Is it tolerable? And most importantly, does it work to improve health?

So, how are clinical trials different from standard care? When your doctor prescribes a medication, they're practicing standard healthcare, not conducting research. Standard therapies are backed by substantial evidence from past clinical trials and are considered standard-of-care only after they have been approved by a regulatory agency such as the **Food and Drug Administration** (FDA) in the United States, and become covered by public (e.g., **Medicare**) or private medical insurance.

Clinical trials are different. They explore new, experimental therapies that often come with many unknowns: Is the drug safe? Does it work? Is it better than what's already available? Usually, several clinical trials are necessary to conclude that an experimental therapy is safe, tolerable, and efficacious. Ultimately, no one will know the outcome until all the trials are done and the data is analyzed. Because of this uncertainty, experimental therapies are not approved by the health regulatory authorities and the cost of the experimental drug used in clinical trials is not covered by medical insurance. If a therapy were already known to be safe, tolerable, and effective, we would not need clinical trials!

Clinical Trials Examine an Intervention

📖 An **intervention** is an action taken on a person or their environment to improve their health. This could involve administering an experimental drug, testing a **medical device**, or implementing a type of psychotherapy.

In most clinical trials, participants are divided into groups that are as similar as possible. Researchers then introduce one or more interventions and carefully monitor the participants, sometimes for years, to assess the intervention's effects.

The most common type of intervention tested in clinical trials is pharmacological: drugs or medications designed to treat specific conditions. These drugs are often novel and experimental, meaning they've never been approved for use before. However, not all interventions involve medications. Non-pharmacological interventions explore alternative ways to improve health without the use of drugs. These include but are not limited to physical therapy, cognitive-behavioral therapy, or lifestyle changes like dietary adjustments. Almost anything can be a clinical trial intervention as long as it is used to investigate its effect on people's health.

🔍 One of the first recorded clinical trials investigated six dietary interventions. In 1747, Scottish physician James Lind, aboard the HMS *Salisbury*, a British naval ship, sought a treatment for scurvy, a devastating disease that plagued sailors on long voyages. At the time, scurvy's cause was unknown, though we now understand it results from a lack of vitamin C, an essential nutrient humans cannot produce and must obtain through diet. Scurvy's symptoms were harrowing: fatigue, muscle pain, swollen and bleeding gums, skin rashes,

Table 1.2 Examples of Clinical Trial Interventions

Intervention	Examples
Pharmacological	Small molecules, hormones, proteins, antibodies, oligonucleotides, viral gene therapies, cell therapies, vaccines
Medical devices	Pacemaker, deep brain stimulation, a phone app
Surgical	Appendectomy, hip replacement
Psychological	Cognitive-behavioral therapy, meditation, psychoanalysis, music therapy
Physical	Physical therapy, yoga, tai-chi, massage
Alternative and complementary	Acupuncture, homeopathy, Chinese traditional medicine
Natural products	Birchbark extract
Diet	Mediterranean diet, low-salt diet
Non-pharmacological	Compression garments, positional changes
Health delivery systems	Face-to-face visits vs. telemedicine. Electronic messaging interventions
Machine learning and artificial intelligence	An algorithm that classifies the severity of patient symptoms in the emergency room
Religious	Prayer

unhealing wounds, and eventually death. Some estimates suggest scurvy caused more deaths during naval expeditions than combat or other diseases, decimating crews and cutting voyages short. Lind's approach to finding a solution was both simple and revolutionary. He divided twelve sailors with scurvy into six groups, providing each group with a different dietary supplement: cider, sulfuric acid, vinegar, seawater, or two citrus fruits (oranges and lemons). For several days, sailors who ate citrus fruits began to recover. Though the link to vitamin C wouldn't be discovered until the twentieth century,

Lind's trial demonstrated that citrus fruits were an effective treatment for scurvy, saving countless lives. While Lind's trial lacked the rigor of modern clinical studies, it was a crucial step in testing interventions systematically in a controlled, comparative manner. Unlike Lind's approach of testing six interventions at once, most modern clinical trials compare just one experimental intervention against a control intervention.

📖 What is a **control intervention**? A control intervention is an intervention that serves as comparison to the new experimental drug. It can take several forms:

- a treatment that is the current **standard of care** for the condition;
- another experimental therapy being tested; or
- a placebo: an intervention with no meaningful biological effect (such as a sugar pill).

📖 What is **randomization**? In most clinical trials, participants are assigned to receive either the active drug or the control intervention through a process called "randomization." This predefined process introduces an element of chance, ensuring the results are unbiased.

I'll dive deeper into the concepts of placebo and randomization in Chapter 2.

Because most clinical trials focus on testing the safety and **efficacy** of experimental drugs, this book will primarily discuss pharmaceutical development. However, it's worth noting that clinical trials aren't limited to medications.

Devices like pacemakers, for example, follow different regulatory approval pathways than drugs. In the United States, the FDA's approval process for new devices can be less rigorous than for drugs. Under the "510(k) pathway," a new device that closely resembles an already approved one (known as a "predicate device") can bypass extensive clinical testing, requiring only evidence of substantial equivalence. While this approach streamlines approval and accelerates patient access to innovative devices, it has raised significant safety concerns. If a predicate device is later found to have defects, any subsequent devices approved based on that predicate could inherit similar risks without rigorous independent testing. For example, faulty hip implants and transvaginal mesh devices (approved through the 510(k) pathway) have led to thousands of patient injuries and costly recalls.[1] This serves as a reminder of the critical balance between innovation and safety in medical device approval.

Clinical Trials Study Human Beings

The third key term in the definition of clinical trials is "human." Studies conducted in animals, microorganisms, or cells, even if they involve interventions, are not considered clinical trials. For example, a placebo-controlled study testing whether an experimental drug improves heart failure in monkeys is a **preclinical** study, not a clinical trial. Even studies using human cells or tissues aren't classified as clinical trials. To qualify as a clinical trial, the study must involve living human participants.

Many clinical trials involve healthy volunteers. Early-phase clinical trials, such as Phase 1 or first-in-human studies, often recruit healthy individuals to assess safety and tolerability before testing the intervention in patients with specific conditions.

Clinical Trials Measure Health-Related Outcomes

The fourth key concept in the definition is "health-related **outcomes**." But what does this mean? In simple terms, clinical trials measure aspects of health to determine the effects of an intervention. Some health-related outcomes are straightforward, such as survival rates (e.g., how long patients live after a treatment) or the number of medical events, like strokes or heart attacks.

Other outcomes are less obvious but equally important. For instance, in patients with lung diseases, increasing lung capacity is a critical outcome because it correlates with better blood oxygenation. Also, changes in specific proteins linked to a disease (i.e., a **biomarker**) may be considered valid health-related outcomes.

In clinical trials testing psychological interventions, outcomes may focus on behavior or emotional well-being, such as the severity of compulsions in patients with obsessive-compulsive disorder, or changes in mood among smokers attempting to quit.

Clinical Trials Measure Safety and Tolerability

Another vital goal of clinical trials is to evaluate the safety and tolerability of an intervention.

📖 **Safety** refers to potential harm, or **adverse effects**, caused by an intervention. These adverse effects can range from mild (e.g., nausea, headaches) to severe (e.g., organ damage, life-threatening reactions).

📖 **Tolerability** focuses on how well participants can handle side effects. For example, while an intervention may be considered safe (not causing life-threatening reactions), severe nausea could make it intolerable for many patients.

Clinical trials use various methods to assess safety and tolerability, including blood and urine laboratory tests, physical examinations, and diverse event monitoring (e.g., tracking side effects reported by participants). The methods vary depending on the intervention. For instance, a psychological therapy trial might not require blood tests but would still monitor for emotional or behavioral side effects.

📖 **Adherence**, also called *compliance*, is another critical factor in clinical trials. This measures how well participants follow study instructions, such as taking medications as directed by researchers. Poor tolerability can often lead to low adherence, which affects study outcomes.

The Risk-Benefit Ratio

Safety and tolerability play a crucial role in determining an intervention's risk-benefit ratio: the balance between potential risks and benefits.

📖 **Risk-benefit ratio**: This evaluation compares the harms (e.g., safety concerns, poor tolerability) of an intervention to its potential benefits on participants' health. A favorable risk-benefit ratio means the benefits outweigh the risks, which is a key factor in advancing a treatment. The more participants tested in clinical trials, the clearer the risk-benefit ratio becomes. The risk-benefit ratio depends on the intervention, the condition being treated, and the availability of other treatments.

The risks and benefits are different for everyone. The willingness to accept risk depends on the severity of the disease (more willingness), duration of treatment (the shorter the duration the more willingness), whether the therapy is preventive (less willingness), or whether the patient group is vulnerable (e.g., pediatric, less willingness).

🔍 Imagine a new experimental drug for glioblastoma multiforme, an aggressive brain cancer with a grim average survival of just fifteen months. The hypothetical drug could extend survival to twenty-seven months (an additional year) but causes severe daily nausea, vomiting, and fatigue. For many glioblastoma patients, the added survival time might outweigh the risks, especially if other available medications can help manage side effects. Now, consider another hypothetical drug for migraines that also causes severe nausea and fatigue. Even if it effectively stops headaches, most migraine patients would likely avoid it. Safer, more tolerable, and widely available options (e.g., ibuprofen or acetaminophen) would be preferable.

Overview of the Clinical Trial Phases

Before a drug can receive regulatory approval, it must demonstrate a positive risk-benefit assessment in humans. This evaluation occurs through a series of clinical trials conducted in distinct phases. Each phase builds on the findings of the previous one, gradually increasing in size, complexity, and scope.

Most clinical trials unfold across three main phases:

- Phase 1: Small-scale safety studies.
- Phase 2: Larger trials to assess safety and early signs of effectiveness.
- Phase 3: Large-scale studies comparing the drug to the current standard treatment or placebo to confirm efficacy.

Table 1.3 Characteristics of the Main Clinical Trial Phases

	Phase 1	Phase 2	Phase 3
Size	20 to 100 participants	100 to 500 participants	200 to 3,000 participants
Duration	1–2 years	1–3 years	3–5 years
Main Goal	Assess safety and most promising dose	Evaluate safety and efficacy	Confirm safety and efficacy

Phase 1: First-in-Human Trials

Phase 1 trials are the first step in testing a drug in humans, earning them the nickname first-in-human trials. These studies, smaller than Phase 2 and Phase 3 trials, primarily aim to evaluate a drug's safety and determine the most promising dosage for future trials. Researchers answer questions like how long the drug stays in the body, what the effects of different doses of the drug are, and if there are any immediate adverse reactions.

Think of Phase 1 as a cautious "first date" between a drug and human volunteers. Researchers proceed carefully, monitoring participants in specialized clinics, sometimes for several days, to ensure the relationship doesn't turn toxic.

Key Facts about Phase 1 Trials:

- Participants: Typically, 20–100 people, often healthy volunteers. However, patients may participate in trials for certain conditions like cancer, neurodegenerative disorders, or rare diseases.

- Focus: Safety, tolerability, and dosage. While Phase 1 trials may use biomarkers (e.g., blood tests or imaging) to hint at efficacy, assessing efficacy is not their primary goal.

- Duration and Cost: Phase 1 trials are relatively short, lasting a few months to a couple of years, and less expensive than later phases, typically costing between several hundred thousand and a few million dollars. Importantly, these costs are covered by the sponsor, not the participants! (For more details on who pays for clinical trials, see the end of this chapter.)

Sometimes, you may see that a trial is labeled Phase 1a. This is the initial first-in-human study, often involving single doses in healthy volunteers. A Phase 1b is a follow-up trial with multiple doses, usually involving patients instead of healthy volunteers.

In terms of success rate, approximately 65 percent of Phase 1 trials progress to Phase 2.[2] In other words, approximately four out of ten compounds tested in a Phase 1 trial fail. Most failures occur due to safety concerns or poor pharmacokinetics.

📖 **Pharmacokinetics (PK):** The study of how a drug moves through the body over time. This includes absorption (how it enters the bloodstream), distribution (how it spreads to different tissues), metabolism (how the body breaks it down), and excretion (how it is eliminated). In simple terms, pharmacokinetics answers the question: What does the body do to the drug?

Phase 2: Assessing Efficacy and Refining Safety

Once a drug is deemed safe in Phase 1, it advances to Phase 2, where researchers focus on evaluating its preliminary efficacy and refining its safety profile in a larger group of patients with the target condition.

Key Facts about Phase 2 trials:

- Participants: Typically, 100–500 patients.
- Focus: Assessing preliminary efficacy, refining the dosage to be used in future trials, and identifying side effects that may not have emerged during Phase 1.
- Duration and Cost: Phase 2 trials usually last one to three years. They cost from a few million to tens of millions of dollars, depending on trial complexity.

Sometimes you may see a trial labeled as a Phase 2a. This is a smaller, less complex study focusing on dosage and safety Conversely, Phase 2b is a larger, more complex study assessing efficacy more rigorously.

In terms of success rates, approximately 48 percent of Phase 2 trials progress to Phase 3. This means nearly half of the compounds tested in Phase 2 fail to advance, primarily due to inadequate efficacy or emerging safety concerns. When we consider the cumulative failure rates from Phase 1 through Phase 2, the outlook becomes even more sobering: out of every ten experimental drugs that begin Phase 1, only about three will make it to Phase 3.

Phase 3: Confirming Safety and Efficacy

If a drug demonstrates promise in Phase 2, it advances to Phase 3, the most extensive and rigorous stage of the clinical trial process. Phase 3 trials aim to confirm the drug's safety and efficacy in a broader population.

Key Facts about Phase 3 Trials:

- Participants: Hundreds to several thousand, depending on disease prevalence and trial design.
- Focus: Comparing the experimental drug to standard treatments or placebo to confirm efficacy and collecting additional safety data to identify rare or long-term side effects.
- Duration and Cost: Phase 3 trials have a typical duration of three to five years. They are significantly more expensive than previous phases, costing tens to hundreds of millions of dollars.

The design of Phase 3 is also more complex; they are often multicenter and multinational, involving diverse populations to assess the drug's effectiveness across different groups.

In terms of success rates, around 59 percent of Phase 3 trials result in regulatory approval.[3] Collectively considering the success rates of Phase 1, Phase 2, and Phase 3 trials, this means only one to two out of every ten drugs initially tested in Phase 1 will ultimately succeed. Sobering, isn't it? The journey from Phase 1 to approval is long, expensive, and uncertain, but it's the foundation of safe, effective medicine.

⚠ Could the same person participate in all three phases? It's generally uncommon for the same participant to take part in Phase 1, Phase 2, and Phase 3 trials of the same experimental therapy, although it's not entirely impossible. Eligibility depends on factors such as inclusion and exclusion criteria (we will discuss these criteria in Chapter 5) and the time gap between phases. For example, the disease stages targeted in each trial may differ, or prior exposure to the drug in earlier trials might disqualify participation in later phases. However, in rare diseases with few patients, sponsors might recruit the same participant across multiple phases to ensure sufficient enrollment.

Other Phases

In addition to the standard Phases 1 to 3, some clinical trials are categorized as Phase 0 or Phase 4, serving distinct purposes in the drug development process.

Phase 0 trials are even smaller than Phase 1 trials, involving fewer than ten participants who receive very low drug doses over short periods. These studies, sometimes conducted in oncology, aim to detect biochemical responses to the drug, even though the doses are too low to provide therapeutic benefit. The main advantage is that the minimal doses carry a very low risk of side effects. The main limitation is that Phase 0 trials are not designed to evaluate efficacy, and any observed effects are preliminary at best.

Phase 4 trials, on the other side of the spectrum, are conducted after a drug has received regulatory approval and is available on the market. While the drug is no longer experimental, these trials are still considered clinical research because they evaluate the drug in broader or specialized populations. Why would someone decide to participate in a Phase 4 trial if the drug is not experimental anymore?

- Early Access: Some Phase 4 trials allow patients to receive the drug before it is widely available in pharmacies.
- Free Access: Patients may receive the drug for free, particularly if insurance coverage is limited.
- Close Monitoring: Participants benefit from frequent check-ins and oversight, which may provide added reassurance when starting a new treatment.

The goals of Phase 4 trials are to detect rare adverse effects, evaluate long-term safety, and study the drug's effectiveness in broader or diverse populations. Phase 4 trials often involve hundreds of thousands, or even millions, of patients worldwide. They are typically part of routine pharmacovigilance programs and can continue for years or decades to monitor the drug's safety profile.

Why So Many Phases?

Wondering why so many phases? It's like building a skyscraper: you need a solid foundation before adding more floors.

This stepwise approach serves multiple purposes. By starting small (e.g., Phase 1 trials), researchers can identify severe side effects early, minimizing risks to larger populations. Each phase builds on the findings of the previous one, ensuring a methodical evaluation of safety and efficacy. Early-phase trials are less expensive and less complex, so resources aren't wasted on drugs that don't show promise.

However, this process has a major drawback: time. Completing all trial phases sequentially can take years or even decades, leaving patients waiting for new therapies.

But, again, this is done in the name of safety. And still, despite the rigorous preclinical testing in animals, rare and catastrophic adverse effects could still occur in Phase 1 human trials, although such events are exceedingly uncommon.

🔍 Devastating accidents in Phase 1 first-in-human trials are extremely rare, but they leave a lasting impression because they often affect healthy young volunteers. The death or serious damage to a group of healthy volunteers is the nightmare each researcher involved in early drug trials fears the most. In 1985, a volunteer died while testing a new heart rhythm medication called eproxindine. In 2006, several volunteers nearly died from a severe immune system overreaction when testing a drug called theralizumab (also known as TGN1412), which was meant to treat certain immune disorders. In 2016, one volunteer died and five others suffered severe brain damage during a trial for BIA-10-2474, an experimental pain medication. These tragic events serve as a stark reminder that despite extensive safety measures, testing new medicines on humans for the first time can still carry unexpected and sometimes dire risks. They underscore the delicate balance between advancing medical science and protecting the well-being of those who volunteer for such trials.

Must All Drugs Complete Every Phase?

Not all experimental drugs need to complete every clinical trial phase. Extraordinary circumstances, such as rare diseases, public health emergencies, or drug repurposing, allow for exceptions.

Public Health Emergencies

During crises like the COVID-19 pandemic, traditional drug development timelines are accelerated. Trials are conducted simultaneously rather than sequentially; trial protocols are modified in real time based on preliminary data; and large-scale vaccine manufacturing begins before regulatory approval to ensure immediate availability.

In the case of COVID-19, in less than a year, vaccines like those from Pfizer-BioNTech and Moderna went from clinical trials to emergency use authorization. This unprecedented speed was made possible through global collaboration, massive funding, and adaptive trial designs (more on adaptive trials in Chapter 9).

Rare Diseases

Rare diseases (sometimes also called **orphan diseases**) affecting fewer than 200,000 people in the United States, often present unique challenges for clinical trials. Recruiting enough patients to complete large-scale trials is impractical, so regulatory agencies may streamline the process by requiring fewer participants or skipping trial phases.

🔍 Spinal muscular atrophy (SMA), a rare and deadly genetic condition affecting infants and young children, causes muscle weakness and often leads to death before age two. The gene therapy Zolgensma® works by providing a working copy of the gene missing in SMA patients, using a harmless virus to deliver it. This helps restore normal protein production in the spinal cord, potentially stopping or even reversing the disease's progress. What makes Zolgensma® remarkable is not just its technology, but how it was tested and approved. The initial trial involved only fifteen babies, with no placebo group. Yet the results were astonishing: almost all treated infants lived past twenty months, a milestone rarely reached by untreated SMA babies without permanent breathing support. These children didn't just survive; they showed significant improvements in movement, with some nearly matching healthy children's development. The

FDA approved Zolgensma® in 2019 based on data from just thirty-six babies, while a larger study was still ongoing. This quick approval offered hope to families who previously had no effective treatment options.

Drug Repurposing

📖 **Drug repurposing** explores new uses for existing medications that are already approved for other conditions. Repurposed drugs skip many early development stages, as their safety and pharmacological properties are already well documented. This can result in shorter timelines and faster approvals, in a cost-effective, more efficient pathway for bringing new therapies to patients.

🔍 In the small English town of Sandwich, Pfizer researchers were studying a compound called sildenafil to treat angina, a condition caused by reduced blood flow to the heart. Early trials showed the drug wasn't effective for angina, but researchers noticed an unexpected side effect: male participants reported improved erectile function. Recognizing the potential, Pfizer pivoted. Sildenafil, branded as Viagra®, became the first FDA-approved oral treatment for erectile dysfunction in 1998. It was a commercial success, generating billions in revenue and becoming a global phenomenon. The blue pill gained widespread attention, with *Time* magazine featuring it on its cover, and the *New York Times* describing it as the most successful drug introduction ever in the United States.

The serendipitous discovery of Viagra® exemplifies the power of repurposing existing drugs. A compound initially tested for heart disease went on to change lives in a completely different way and cemented its place in medical history. Other examples of repurposed drugs are aspirin (originally a pain reliever, now used to prevent heart attacks and stroke), finasteride (first approved for prostate enlargement, later repurposed for hair loss) and sunitinib (first approved for renal cell carcinoma, later approved for pancreatic tumors).

Overview of the Drug Development Process

While clinical trials are the centerpiece of drug development, they are just one stage in a complex process. Multiple steps must occur before and after clinical trials for a healthcare provider to be able to prescribe a new drug. Developing a new drug is a monumental endeavor, costing an estimated $1–2 billion and often taking over a decade.[4] Here's a closer look at the stages that bring a new medicine from the lab to the public.

Drug Discovery and Research

The journey begins with identifying potential drug candidates. Scientists explore biological mechanisms, identify therapeutic targets, and conduct experiments to find molecules that could become future drugs. The targets could be a gene, protein, enzyme, or other molecule linked to a disease. For example, a receptor involved in cancer growth might become a target for a drug that blocks its activity. Scientists then search for molecules that interact with the target using techniques like high-throughput screening or computational modeling. These molecules can come from natural sources, existing drugs, or be newly synthesized in laboratories. Once promising candidates are identified, they undergo chemical optimization to improve their potency, selectivity, pharmacokinetics, and safety.

🔍 Japanese scientist Akira Endo discovered the first statin, mevastatin, after screening molds and fungi for compounds that could lower cholesterol. One of his most promising finds came from an unexpected place: a blue-green mold growing on a bag of rice in a Kyoto grain shop. His work eventually led to the development of statins like simvastatin (Zocor®) and atorvastatin (Lipitor®), which became lifesaving drugs for millions.

Preclinical Testing

Before testing in humans, potential drugs undergo extensive laboratory and animal studies. The goals of preclinical testing are to determine if the drug causes toxicity or harmful side effects, study how the drug is absorbed, distributed, metabolized, and excreted, and gather preliminary evidence that the drug can achieve its intended effect. Animal studies also test fertility, pregnancy safety, and the potential for genetic damage or birth defects. The data collected informs decisions about whether a drug is ready for human trials and helps design those trials.

Clinical Development

The clinical development phase consists of human trials (discussed in detail earlier in this chapter). These trials evaluate safety, efficacy, and dosing, often requiring years of effort and significant financial investment.

Regulatory Review

Once Phase 3 trials are completed, the sponsor compiles the data into a dossier and submits it to regulatory agencies like the FDA. This submission includes results from preclinical studies, clinical trials, and proposed labeling for the drug. The regulatory agency will then scrutinize the data for safety and efficacy, seek input from patient advocacy groups and expert panels, and decide whether the drug can be approved or whether additional data is required.

🔍 The modern FDA owes its prominence to a tragedy in the 1930s when "Elixir Sulfanilamide" (a drug dissolved in toxic diethylene glycol) caused more than seventy deaths, including many children. The scandal prompted the passage of the 1938 Federal Food, Drug, and Cosmetic Act, requiring drugs to be proven safe before marketing. Today, the FDA approves twenty to forty new drugs annually. In 2023, it approved fifty-six drugs, including treatments for cancer, neurology, infectious diseases, and even a birchbark extract.

Approval and Market Access

Once approved, the drug enters the market, but the journey isn't over. The drug must receive a proprietary name (e.g., Motrin® or Advil®) alongside its pharmacological name (ibuprofen). Pharmaceutical companies negotiate prices with Medicare and insurance providers, which will cover most of the drug's cost. Finally, the drug is shipped to pharmacies, making it accessible to patients.

Even after approval, a drug may be withdrawn if a safer or more effective treatment becomes available, or post-market safety monitoring reveals serious risks. While the system is designed to safeguard patients, it's not perfect.

🔍 Rofecoxib, developed by Merck, was a COX-2 inhibitor approved in 1999 to relieve pain and inflammation with fewer gastrointestinal side effects than traditional painkillers like ibuprofen. It was widely prescribed, with more than 80 million users worldwide. In 2004, Merck voluntarily withdrew Vioxx® after studies revealed an increased risk of heart attack and stroke with long-term, high-dose use. Investigations estimated that the drug had caused approximately 150,000 heart attacks, half of which were fatal. Merck faced numerous lawsuits. The Vioxx® controversy prompted stricter regulatory measures, including enhanced cardiovascular safety testing, more rigorous post-market surveillance, and improved **adverse event** reporting standards. These reforms were designed to prevent similar tragedies and strengthen patient safety.

Who Is Responsible and Pays for a Clinical Trial?

The responsibilities in a clinical trial are shared between two key players: the sponsor and the principal investigator (PI).

📖 The **sponsor** is the organization that initiates and oversees the clinical trial. Think of the sponsor as the orchestra conductor, coordinating all elements of the trial to ensure smooth execution. Pharmaceutical and **biotechnology** companies are the most frequent sponsors, providing the funding needed for drug manufacturing, testing, and logistical expenses. Academic institutions, research hospitals, or government agencies may sponsor smaller trials, particularly investigator-initiated trials.

📖 The **principal investigator (PI)** is the qualified physician or researcher responsible for conducting the trial at a specific site. If a trial is conducted at multiple sites, each site will have its local PI. The PI acts as the ship's captain, leading the trial team (e.g., other **investigators**, **research coordinators**, and research nurses), ensures participant safety and adherence to the trial **protocol**, and reports any safety issues to the sponsor. While the sponsor holds ultimate responsibility for the trial, the PI is critical in safeguarding participants and ensuring ethical conduct at the site level.

⚠ Watch out for double-dipping. Sponsors are required to cover all trial-related expenses, including procedures and assessments.

However, some institutions engage in illegal "double-dipping" by billing health insurance for procedures already paid for by the sponsor. Such fraudulent behavior is punishable by law with hefty fines, and its occurrence is not restricted to small, shady medical offices.

🔍 In January 2024, the prestigious H. Lee Moffitt Cancer Center & Research Institute in Tampa, Florida, agreed to pay $19.5 million to resolve allegations of improper billing for clinical trial costs. The settlement arose after the cancer center improperly billed Medicare and Medicaid for clinical trial expenses that had been already paid for by trial sponsors. The billing irregularities spanned six years, from 2014 to 2020, and involved claims for clinical trial-related procedures that failed to meet the strict guidelines set by the Centers for Medicare and Medicaid Services (CMS). While Moffitt's steps mitigated the penalties, this case serves as a powerful reminder of the importance of transparency and adherence to regulations in clinical research.

Who Oversees Clinical Trials?

Clinical trials are tightly regulated and monitored to ensure participant safety, scientific integrity, and ethical conduct. Several key groups oversee clinical trials, each with distinct roles.

Regulatory Agencies: The Gatekeepers of Drug Development

Before a clinical trial can begin, it must be approved by a regulatory agency, which ensures that the study meets legal and ethical standards. In the United States, this is the FDA, while in Europe, it's the European Medicines Agency (EMA). These agencies evaluate whether a proposed clinical trial is scientifically sound, assess the risks and benefits of new drugs, and ultimately decide whether a treatment can be approved and marketed to the public.

But their oversight doesn't stop once a trial begins; regulatory agencies continue to monitor ongoing trials, reviewing safety data, approving protocol changes, and even halting studies if risks outweigh benefits.

Institutional Review Boards (IRBs) and Ethics Committees: Protecting Participants

Regulatory agencies set broad guidelines, but **institutional review boards (IRBs)**, also known as Ethics Committees outside the United States, act as local ethical watchdogs. Every clinical trial protocol must have IRB approval before enrolling participants at each of the research sites. In other words, without IRB approval, a trial cannot move forward. IRBs are responsible for protecting the rights, safety, and well-being of trial participants by ensuring the study is ethically sound and scientifically justified.

Not all IRBs are the same. Depending on the type of study, where it's conducted, and funding sources, a trial may be reviewed by one or more of the following:

- Academic (Institutional) IRBs: These are housed within universities, medical schools, or hospitals conducting research. They typically review trials run by their own faculty and researchers.

- Commercial (Independent) IRBs: These are private, for-profit organizations that review trials independently of any university or hospital. These IRBs are commonly used for industry-sponsored (pharmaceutical) trials because they are faster than academic IRBs (less red tape), and have more experience in handling multisite, international trials.

- Centralized IRBs: These are used for multisite trials, where one IRB oversees research at multiple institutions instead of requiring each site to get separate approval. This streamlines review, reduces duplication, and ensures consistent ethical oversight across all locations. However, academic institutions may still require their local IRBs to sign off (slowing down the process).

IRBs evaluate a trial's risks and benefits, focusing on key issues such as:

- Informed consent: Is the information on the informed consent form clear, transparent, and free from coercion? (More about the informed consent process in Chapter 5.)
- Risk minimization: Are participants exposed to unnecessary harm (e.g., too many biopsies)?
- Privacy and confidentiality: Are patient records properly protected?

Most IRBs meet regularly to review new trials and monitor ongoing studies. If a trial has significant risks, IRBs may require more frequent updates, participant check-ins, or even halt the trial if safety concerns arise.

Data Safety Monitoring Board (DSMB): The Independent Watchdog

Some trials, especially large, high-risk, or long-term studies, require an additional layer of oversight: a **Data Safety Monitoring Board (DSMB)**. This is an independent panel of experts (clinicians, statisticians, and researchers) who review trial data in real time to:

- detect unexpected safety concerns before they become serious;

- determine if the trial should continue, be modified, or be stopped early; and
- ensure the trial remains scientifically valid.

Unlike IRBs, DSMBs have access to ongoing, unblinded data (i.e., they can see which participants received the drug vs. placebo), allowing them to identify problems before they become public health risks.

Other Oversight Committees: Specialized Review Panels

Depending on the study, additional committees may be involved. For instance, some trials have "adjudication committees" comprising independent experts who confirm diagnoses and endpoints to ensure trial data is reliable; other trials have a "steering committee," a group of senior investigators who provide advice and help guide complex trials.

Clinical trials operate under a multilayered safety net of regulatory agencies, IRBs, DSMBs, and other oversight committees. This system exists to protect participants while ensuring that new treatments are backed by rigorous, ethical, and transparent science.

Ten Clinical Trials Myths

There are many misconceptions about clinical trials. Let's address some of the most common ones.

Myth #1: Only terminal patients qualify for trials. While some trials do focus on patients with advanced or treatment-resistant conditions, many also include individuals in earlier stages of disease, those with stable conditions, or even healthy volunteers (e.g., Phase 1 trials). Trials for preventive care, early detection, or symptom management often involve people who are not critically ill. For instance, clinical trials for cholesterol-lowering medications like statins involved participants with high cholesterol levels but no history of heart attacks. Similarly, vaccine trials often recruit healthy individuals to test their safety and efficacy. Even if your condition is stable or well controlled, a clinical trial could offer an opportunity to explore innovative treatments.

Myth #2: Clinical trials only test cutting-edge experimental drugs. Trials often test existing drugs for new indications, dosages, or delivery methods. For example, aspirin was originally tested as a pain reliever before trials revealed its benefits for preventing heart attacks and stroke.

Myth #3: You're just a "guinea pig" in a clinical trial. Participants are not test subjects in the traditional sense. Clinical trials are carefully designed to prioritize safety, ethics, and informed consent. Preclinical testing in animals minimizes risks before a drug reaches human trials, and participants are monitored closely throughout the study.

Myth #4: Placebo means no treatment. While some participants in trials receive a placebo (an inactive substance), many trials compare a new drug to the standard of care. Even in placebo-controlled trials, participants are monitored closely and may receive better overall care than they would outside the trial.

Myth #5: Once you enroll, you can't leave a clinical trial. Participation in clinical trials is completely voluntary. You can withdraw at any time for any reason (or even for no reason!) without facing penalties or losing access to standard medical care.

Myth #6: Clinical trials are always unsafe. While clinical trials inherently involve some level of risk, every precaution is taken to ensure participant safety. Trials must follow strict regulatory guidelines and are monitored by ethics committees, IRBs, and regulatory agencies like the FDA.

Myth #7: Clinical trials are only available in big cities. While many trials are conducted in large research hospitals or academic institutions, smaller hospitals, clinics, and even community centers often run trials. Additionally, **decentralized clinical trials** are becoming more common, allowing participants to complete parts of the study remotely (more on decentralized trials in Chapter 9).

Myth #8: Only younger people can participate. Many trials specifically target older adults, particularly for diseases like Alzheimer's, Parkinson's, and arthritis. Age requirements depend on the trial and its objectives, but older populations are often included in studies for chronic and age-related conditions.

Myth #9: Clinical trials are always time consuming. While some trials require frequent visits or intensive participation, others involve minimal time commitments. Most trials offer compensation for time and travel expenses, and remote options are increasingly available.

Myth #10: Participating in a trial means you're guaranteed to get the experimental drug. Everyone in a trial may not receive the experimental treatment. Depending on the trial design, some participants may receive a placebo or standard-of-care treatment to allow researchers to make comparisons.

Chapter 1 Highlights

- Clinical trials are research studies involving human participants, designed to evaluate the effects of interventions (e.g., new drugs) on health outcomes.
- A key objective of clinical trials is to assess the safety and tolerability of experimental therapies and determine whether their benefits outweigh the risks.
- Clinical trials for new drugs typically proceed through three main phases (Phases 1 to 3), although their duration and structure can vary depending on the drug and disease under investigation.
- Drug development is a costly and lengthy process, with clinical trials serving as one critical stage in a much broader effort.
- Distinguishing between legitimate clinical trials and scams is essential to protect patients and caregivers.
- The sponsor (often a pharmaceutical company, academic institution, or research organization) is responsible for funding and overseeing the trial.

Notes

1. These issues are highlighted in the documentary *The Bleeding Edge* (available on Netflix), which explores the potential consequences of these regulatory gaps.
2. Chi Heem Wong, Kien Wei Siah, and Andrew W. Lo, "Estimation of Clinical Trial Success Rates and Related Parameters," *Biostatistics* 20, no. 2 (April 2019): 273–86.

3   Ibid.

4   Olivier J. Wouters, Martin McKee, Jeroen Luyten, et al., "Estimated Research and Development Investment Needed to Bring a New Medicine to Market, 2009–2018," *Journal of the American Medical Association* 323, no. 9 (March 2020): 844–53.

2

Should You Join a Clinical Trial?

Deciding whether to join a clinical trial is one of the most important, and often daunting, choices a patient or caregiver may face. It's not just a medical decision but an emotional, ethical, and deeply personal one.

Clinical trials are often painted as a beacon of hope for those with limited options, offering access to cutting-edge therapies and the chance to contribute to advancing science. Yet, participating in a clinical trial is not without challenges or risks. Participating in a trial requires a significant commitment, a level of comfort with uncertainty, and an understanding that the experimental drug may not be safe or effective. Volunteers may receive a placebo instead of the experimental drug, experience unexpected side effects, or find that the therapy simply doesn't work. Just like investing in the stock market, participants need to be prepared for the possibility that things may not work out as they had wished. In addition, trials often demand significant commitments, frequent hospital visits, hours-long questionnaires, or uncomfortable procedures like repeated blood draws.

Clinical trials aren't for everyone. Not everyone is willing or able to accept these uncertainties, and that's fine. Ultimately, the decision to participate in a clinical trial is profoundly personal, shaped by individual circumstances, risk tolerance, and values.

In this chapter, I'll go over these hurdles and break down key concepts like placebo and randomization, the major risks you may face as a clinical trial participant, as well as practical advice on discussing trials with your doctor. Armed with knowledge, you'll be better prepared to make an informed choice and decide if clinical trials are the right option for you or your loved one.

The Good, the Bad, and the Ugly: Real-World Cases of Extreme Success or Failure

Clinical trials are transformative but complex, with outcomes ranging from life-changing success to heartbreaking failure. To help you understand the stakes, here are real-world examples of clinical trial participants whose stories illustrate the extreme possibilities of trial outcomes. While these stories highlight extraordinary cases, they reflect the spectrum of experiences you may encounter.

The Good

🔍 Emily Whitehead, diagnosed with an aggressive form of leukemia at age five, faced dire odds after traditional treatments failed. In 2012, she became the first pediatric patient to receive chimeric antigen receptor (CAR) T-cell therapy in a clinical trial at Children's Hospital of Philadelphia. CAR T-cell therapy involves modifying a patient's immune cells to target cancer. The treatment was not without risks. Emily developed severe side effects, including the life-threatening "cytokine release syndrome," a complication of CAR T-cell therapy.

However, her care team quickly intervened with an anti-inflammatory drug, which saved her life. Amazingly, Emily's cancer went into complete remission, and it has stayed that way ever since. As of today, she is thriving, a testament to the groundbreaking potential of clinical trials. Her case highlights how trials can pave the way for revolutionary treatments and offer a second chance at life for patients with few options left.

The Bad

🔍 Jesse Gelsinger was an outgoing and adventurous eighteen-year-old from Tucson, Arizona, living with ornithine transcarbamylase (OTC) deficiency, a rare genetic disorder that prevents the body from properly eliminating ammonia, a toxic byproduct of protein metabolism. Jesse's condition was a milder form of the disorder, allowing him to manage it through a strict diet and medication. In 1999, Jesse volunteered for a groundbreaking gene therapy trial at the University of Pennsylvania. The experimental therapy aimed to replace the faulty OTC gene with a functional one, delivered using an adenoviral vector (a modified virus designed to transport genetic material into cells). However, shortly after receiving the therapy, Jesse experienced a catastrophic immune reaction, resulting in multiple organ failure and brain death. Four days later, on September 17, 1999, Jesse's parents made the agonizing decision to remove him from life support. Jesse was the first person known to die in a gene therapy trial, sending shockwaves through the scientific community. His death raised serious questions about trial safety, informed consent, and regulatory oversight, leading to stricter guidelines for clinical research. Jesse's tragic experience became a turning point in gene therapy research, reminding the world of the profound responsibilities owed to clinical trial participants.

🔍 Terry Horgan, a twenty-seven-year-old from Montclair, New Jersey, lived with Duchenne muscular dystrophy (DMD), a genetic disorder characterized by progressive muscle degeneration. Caused by mutations in the dystrophin gene, DMD primarily affects boys and often leads to loss of mobility, respiratory complications, and early death. In 2022, Terry joined a clinical trial for an experimental viral gene therapy designed to replace the defective dystrophin gene with a synthetic, functional version, with the goal of halting or even reversing the progression of DMD. For Terry and many others living with the disorder, the therapy represented a glimmer of hope. Tragically, just a few weeks after receiving the therapy, Terry developed severe complications, including heart inflammation and multi-organ failure, and passed away on June 30, 2022. His death was particularly devastating for his brother, Rich, who had dedicated his life to finding a cure for DMD by founding Cure Rare Disease, the organization that sponsored the trial.

Both Jesse Gelsinger and Terry Horgan were young men full of hope, volunteering not just for themselves, but for the advancement of medical science. Their untimely deaths were heartbreaking reminders of the risks inherent in clinical trials, particularly for experimental therapies. However, their legacies live on: Jesse's case led to sweeping reforms in trial safety, while Terry's inspires continued efforts to develop therapies for devastating rare diseases like DMD.

The Ugly

🔍 Josh Hardy was a brave seven-year-old boy from Fredericksburg, Virginia, who had already faced more medical challenges in his short life than many experience in a lifetime. After surviving kidney cancer and enduring intensive chemotherapy, Josh underwent a bone marrow transplant to address complications from his treatment.

While the transplant was initially successful, Josh developed a life-threatening adenoviral infection, which standard treatments could not control. In a desperate attempt to save their son, Josh's parents learned of brincidofovir, an experimental antiviral drug being developed by the small pharmaceutical company Chimerix. The drug was still in clinical trials and had not been approved for general use, but Josh's family was determined to get him access. They requested the "compassionate use" of the drug, which would allow Josh to receive it outside the trial (we will go over the concept of compassionate use in detail in Chapter 3). However, Chimerix initially denied the request, citing concerns about the safety and efficacy of the unproven drug, as well as the limited supply available for the then-ongoing trials. This decision ignited a storm of public outrage. Josh's family launched a viral social media campaign under the hashtag #SaveJosh, accusing Chimerix and its CEO of prioritizing corporate interests over saving a child's life. The hashtag quickly gained traction, becoming a trending topic, while national media outlets covered the story daily. The campaign garnered massive support from celebrities, politicians, and ordinary citizens who rallied behind the Hardy family. Amid mounting pressure and widespread condemnation, including thousands of phone calls, emails, and even death threats directed at the CEO, Chimerix worked with the FDA to grant Josh access to the drug. Initially, his health seemed to improve. For a brief time, it appeared the drug was working. However, the relief was short-lived. The adenovirus returned, and Josh passed away later that year, succumbing to complications related to the infection.

The aftermath of Josh's death was just as tragic as his journey. Subsequent clinical trials revealed that brincidofovir was ineffective in treating adenovirus. Despite showing promise in early preclinical studies, the drug failed to demonstrate any meaningful benefit when tested in humans. What Josh's parents, and many who participated in the emotional social media frenzy, had believed to be a "miracle cure" ultimately turned out to be a drug failure.

This case raised complex questions. Josh's parents were driven by a desperate love for their son and a natural desire to do whatever it took to save him. But their relentless efforts to bypass the trial system not only left Josh vulnerable but also contributed to a societal backlash against a biotech company that tried to maintain a delicate balance of ethics, safety, and scientific rigor while developing an experimental drug that turned out to be ineffective. The case also highlights the need for better education about clinical trial processes, ensuring patients and their families can make informed decisions when this matters the most.

The stories of Emily, Terry, Jesse, and Josh highlight the highs and lows of clinical trials. The good is that clinical trials can lead to groundbreaking therapies, transforming lives like Emily Whitehead's. The bad is that they also carry risks, as shown by Jesse Gelsinger's case, where unforeseen complications can have tragic outcomes. Sometimes, ugly situations occur when, even with good intentions, some try to find loopholes in the clinical trial process. These cases are not just cautionary tales; they are reminders that participating in a clinical trial is a deeply personal decision requiring careful consideration of the potential benefits, risks, and uncertainties.

Why People Participate in Clinical Trials

The decision to participate in a clinical trial is often motivated by a combination of potential benefits and a desire to contribute to scientific progress. While clinical trials carry potential risks, many participants find the opportunities they provide, both for themselves and others, compelling and worthwhile.

In 2023, a survey by the Center for Information and Study on Clinical Research Participation (CISCRP) found that 96 percent of clinical trial participants would be willing (or somewhat willing) to participate in a clinical trial again. Also, 81 percent of respondents answered that their participation in a clinical trial met or exceeded their expectations, highlighting the positive experiences of joining a clinical trial.[1]

The potential advantages vary depending on the study itself and, importantly, which arm of the study participants are assigned to. For those randomized to the **control group**, the benefits may include receiving the current standard of care, which is often covered at no cost. Participants in any group often gain access to additional monitoring, medical tests, and evaluations that might not otherwise be part of routine care.

Beyond medical benefits, trials can provide intangible rewards: the chance to be more engaged in managing one's health, the camaraderie of connecting with other trial participants facing similar medical challenges, and the knowledge that one's participation could help answer critical questions and improve treatment options for future patients. Ultimately, clinical trials offer a unique opportunity to play an active role in advancing medicine while also receiving care that is often at the cutting edge of science. Let's explore each of these aspects in more detail.

Access to Cutting-Edge Treatments

One of the main advantages of participating in clinical trials is that they can offer an opportunity to access innovative treatments that are not yet widely available. For patients with conditions that lack effective therapies, trials can offer hope where none previously existed.

For example, in the early 2000s, patients with chronic myeloid leukemia who participated in trials for imatinib (Gleevec®) gained access to a groundbreaking drug that transformed a once-fatal disease into a manageable chronic condition. While there are no guarantees that the experimental treatment will work, participation provides a chance to receive the latest advancements in medical science years before they reach the market.

High-Quality Medical Care

Participants in clinical trials often receive state-of-the-art medical care, sometimes at leading research centers. This includes regular monitoring, comprehensive evaluations, and access to expert healthcare professionals specializing in their condition. For instance, a patient in a trial for a new Alzheimer's drug may benefit from detailed, cutting-edge brain imaging and cognitive testing, tests that might otherwise be difficult or expensive to obtain. Moreover, participants get to meet research professionals with whom they establish contact to enrich their knowledge of their disease.

Contributing to Medical Knowledge

By enrolling in a trial, participants play a pivotal role in advancing medical research. Every data point collected (whether the treatment succeeds or has no effect) adds to the collective understanding of a disease and how it can be treated.

Take, for example, the rapid development of COVID-19 vaccines during the pandemic. The willingness of tens of thousands of participants to enroll in clinical trials enabled researchers to evaluate the safety and efficacy of vaccines, saving millions of lives globally. Knowing that their involvement could pave the way for future treatments is a powerful motivator for many participants, especially those with rare diseases who hope to improve options for others like them.

Personalized Health Insights

Participation often involves comprehensive assessments, including lab tests, imaging studies, and detailed medical histories. These evaluations may uncover underlying health issues that the participants may not have known about or provide participants with a clearer understanding of their condition.

For instance, a trial participant with hypertension might receive advanced blood pressure monitoring and tailored feedback on their health. In other cases, the detailed medical assessments required for clinical trials can uncover undiagnosed conditions. For instance, a participant could discover they had an asymptomatic heart arrhythmia thanks to the ECG performed as part of the trial. Identifying this condition early could allow them to receive lifesaving treatments unrelated to the trial.

A Sense of Empowerment and Hope

For many, joining a clinical trial is an act of empowerment, a proactive step in the face of uncertainty. It can provide a sense of control and purpose, particularly for patients with serious illnesses who want to take an active role in their care. Participants can experience a feeling of hopefulness, knowing they are helping themselves while potentially contributing to a future cure or breakthrough for others.

Potential Financial Benefits

Most clinical trials cover trial-related costs, including the experimental treatment, diagnostic tests, and procedures. Some trials also offer reimbursement for travel and other expenses or provide modest compensation for participants' time and effort.

Understanding Potential Clinical Trial Risks and Burdens

While clinical trials can provide opportunities and many potential rewards, they are not without risks. Before deciding to participate, it's essential to understand these risks and how they can be managed. This transparency allows you to weigh the potential benefits against the challenges and uncertainties.

The Risk of Side Effects or Adverse Events

Experimental treatments, by definition, have unknown safety profiles. While preclinical studies and early-phase trials aim to identify major safety concerns, unexpected side effects can still occur when treatments are tested in larger and more diverse populations. For instance, Jesse Gelsinger's story (discussed earlier in this chapter) is a sobering example. In his trial, an experimental gene therapy triggered a severe immune response that led to his tragic death. Such extreme reactions are rare, but milder side effects, like nausea, headache, or fatigue, are common in many trials.

To mitigate this risk, clinical trials include close monitoring of participants to detect side effects early. Regular assessments, such as blood tests or imaging, are designed to catch adverse events before they become severe. Moreover, participants have the right to withdraw from a trial at any time if side effects become intolerable or concerning.

💡 Pro Tip: If you're concerned about safety risks, consider the trial phase. Drugs being tested in Phase 3 trials, for example, often have more extensive safety data compared to those being evaluated in Phase 1 trials, where uncertainty is higher.

The Risk of the Experimental Treatment Not Working

There is no guarantee that the experimental treatment will be effective. Even in promising trials, some participants may experience no benefit, and in some cases, the treatment might worsen their condition. For example, trials testing new Alzheimer's treatments often focus on slowing cognitive decline. A participant might hope for stabilization or improvement, but the experimental drug might fail to produce noticeable results or could even lead to unexpected worsening cognition.

To mitigate this risk, researchers communicate the uncertainty of outcomes during the informed consent process (more on the informed consent process in Chapter 5). Also, clinical trials often include interim analyses (i.e., statistical analyses performed while the trial is still being conducted), allowing researchers to stop the study early if the treatment shows no benefit or poses undue harm.

The Risk of Receiving a Placebo

In placebo-controlled trials, participants might receive a placebo instead of the experimental treatment. We will dive deeper into what a placebo is in the next section, but for, now, you should know that, while placebos are critical for evaluating the treatment's true effects, they can be disappointing or frustrating for participants hoping for relief. For example, in a trial testing a new pain medication, participants in the placebo group might continue to experience discomfort throughout the study.

To mitigate this risk, trials are designed to ensure a fair comparison, often randomizing participants evenly between placebo and treatment groups. Some trials are followed by an open-label extension (OLE) phase, allowing all participants to receive the experimental treatment after the trial ends, provided it is deemed safe (more information on OLE studies in Chapter 7).

⚠ Some participants assume they'll continue receiving the experimental treatment after the trial concludes, especially if it seems to be helping. However, this is not always the case. Access to the drug often ends when the trial is over, as researchers need to analyze the results and gain regulatory approval before the treatment can become widely available. An OLE is never guaranteed.

The Risk of Invasive or Uncomfortable Procedures

Some trials require frequent testing or procedures that may be invasive, uncomfortable, or time consuming. These might include blood draws, spinal taps, biopsies, imaging scans, or hours-long cognitive tests. For instance, in some cancer trials, to monitor the drug's effects participants may undergo repeated bone marrow biopsies, an invasive and often painful procedure.

To mitigate this risk, researchers aim to minimize unnecessary tests and procedures. Participants are informed about all study requirements upfront, allowing them to decide if they are comfortable with the commitment.

The Risk of Time and Travel Burdens

Participating in a clinical trial often requires multiple visits to the study site, which can be a major challenge for individuals with busy schedules or those who live far from research centers. According to a 2023 *Perceptions and Insights Study* conducted by CISCRP, 30 percent of over 4,500 clinical trial participants cited travel to the study site as the most burdensome aspect of participation.[2] While most reported travel times between thirty minutes and one hour, some faced commutes of three hours or more.

Additionally, 36 percent of participants stated that reducing travel distance would have made trial participation significantly less disruptive. These findings underscore how logistical barriers, particularly time and travel demands, can impact patient engagement in clinical research.

To mitigate this, many trials offer financial compensation for travel expenses or provide support for accommodation. Increasingly, decentralized clinical trials allow participants to complete some assessments from home, using virtual telemedicine visits or local facilities. For example, a trial testing a new diabetes treatment could allow participants to submit glucose readings via a smartphone app and have blood samples collected by visiting nurses. These innovations reduce logistical hurdles and make trials more accessible to people with demanding schedules or limited mobility.

The Risk of Financial Costs

Although clinical trials typically cover the cost of the experimental treatment and study-related procedures, participants might face indirect costs, such as travel expenses, lost wages, or childcare.

To prevent this, make sure you ask the trial staff for a clear breakdown of covered costs before enrolling. Also, look for trials that offer stipends or reimbursements for participation-related expenses (more details on clinical trial-related costs in Chapter 6).

The Risk of Emotional and Psychological Stress

Trials can be emotionally taxing, particularly if the treatment doesn't work or if side effects occur. Additionally, the uncertainty of being in a trial can be stressful for participants and their families.

For example, a parent enrolling their child in a pediatric trial might feel anxious about potential risks or guilty if the treatment doesn't help.

To mitigate this risk, some clinical trials include access to counseling or psychological support for participants and their families. Participants should also build a strong support system of friends, family, or patient advocacy groups to help navigate the emotional challenges (more details on how to build support systems during a trial in Chapter 6).

Placebo, Blinding, Randomization, and Other Uncertainties

Clinical trials are designed to answer crucial questions about the safety and efficacy of new treatments, but they often come with layers of uncertainty. This uncertainty is not just a necessary part of the process; it is the foundation of how trials ensure that their findings are unbiased, reliable, and meaningful.

To better understand this, let's explore the roles of placebo, **blinding**, randomization, and other key elements that make clinical trials both robust and, sometimes, challenging for participants.

Placebo: More Than Just a Sugar Pill

📖 A **placebo** is a substance or treatment crafted to resemble the experimental drug in appearance and administration but lacks any direct pharmacological effect. Contrary to some misconceptions, placebos could induce symptomatic benefits; however, these effects stem not from direct pharmacological action on the targeted receptor or condition, but from complex neurobiological mechanisms involving the activation of anticipation, expectation, and reward circuits in the brain, rather than any inherent pharmacological properties of the placebo itself.

The term placebo has a fascinating etymology that reflects its evolving meaning over centuries.[3] Originally, placebo is the first-person singular future indicative of the Latin verb *placere*, meaning "to please." It translates as "I will please." Its usage can be traced back to Psalm 116 in the Latin Vulgate Bible, which contains the verse, "Placebo Domino in regione vivorum" ("I will please the Lord in the land of the living"). This psalm was part of the "Office of the Dead," a set of Catholic prayers offered for the souls of the deceased. By the fourteenth century, "placebo" acquired a cultural association with paid mourners at funerals, individuals hired to please the deceased's family by faking exaggerated grief. Over time, the term expanded to mean someone who offers insincere flattery or false praise (i.e., a sycophant). It wasn't until the late eighteenth century that placebo became a medical term. According to the 1785 *New Medical Dictionary*, "placebo" referred to treatments intended to gratify or soothe a patient, often without therapeutic efficacy. This marked the beginning of its modern usage in medicine as something that mimics treatment to serve as a control in clinical trials or to provide comfort through suggestion rather than active ingredients.

In clinical trials, placebos play a crucial role in helping researchers determine whether the observed beneficial effects of a treatment are truly due to the drug itself or simply the patient's belief that they are receiving effective treatment, a phenomenon known as the "placebo effect." Conversely, the "nocebo effect" arises when a patient's expectation that a drug will cause harm leads to the experience of negative symptoms, even if the treatment itself is harmless.

For example, if an experimental drug is claimed to relieve pain, researchers must determine whether the relief is genuinely caused by the drug's action or if it results from the patient's expectation that they are being treated. The placebo effect can be particularly powerful in certain conditions, such as Parkinson's disease, pain disorders, and psychiatric disorders. In fact, groundbreaking research on Parkinson's disease has shown that when patients are given a placebo under the label of an effective drug, their brains release dopamine, the neurotransmitter that is deficient in Parkinson's, leading to improved symptoms. This demonstrates that the placebo effect is not merely psychological and that it sometimes has real, measurable effects on the body. By comparing the outcomes of participants receiving the experimental drug versus those receiving the placebo, researchers can isolate the true biological effects of the drug from those that might be influenced by the patient's belief or expectation.

To ensure trial results are unbiased, a placebo must resemble the active treatment as closely as possible. This can sometimes be surprisingly complex. For example, if a drug has a noticeable side effect, like staining the urine red, the placebo must also cause this effect to prevent participants from guessing which treatment they are receiving. Without this, the trial could be "unblinded," undermining its integrity.

In trials involving surgical procedures, the placebo arm often uses a **sham procedure**, where participants undergo a modified or partial version of the surgery. For example, in a trial testing a new knee surgery, participants in the placebo group might receive an incision and some minor manipulation of the knee but no actual therapeutic intervention. That's right: they will get a scar despite receiving no treatment. This approach helps ensure that any improvement is due to the experimental surgery itself, not the participants' belief that they were treated.

While placebos are invaluable in many trials, there are situations where their use may be unethical. For instance, when an effective and approved treatment already exists for the condition being studied, it would be unethical to withhold it from participants. In such cases, the control group should receive the standard-of-care treatment rather than a placebo. In a trial testing a new cancer therapy, participants in the control arm might receive the best available chemotherapy regimen to ensure they are not deprived of potentially lifesaving treatment. Similarly, in rapidly progressive diseases with dismal survival rates, it might also be unethical to give patients a placebo. In these situations, any improvement in survival that exceeds what is already known for the disease can be reliably attributed directly to the experimental drug. This was the case with Zolgensma®, the gene therapy for SMA, as discussed in Chapter 1. With survival for babies with severe SMA often measured in a few months, giving a placebo in a trial would have provided no meaningful benefit to participants while exposing them to unnecessary risks.

While placebos can be frustrating for participants who may not receive the active treatment, they are crucial for distinguishing real effects from those driven by expectation. By carefully designing placebo arms and ensuring ethical standards, researchers can uphold the scientific rigor necessary for developing effective therapies while minimizing harm to participants.

Blinding: Keeping Participants (and Researchers) in the Dark

In a blinded trial, participants do not know whether they are receiving the experimental treatment or a placebo. In a **double-blinded** trial, neither the participants nor the researchers administering the treatments know which group the participant belongs to. In some cases, trials are even triple-blinded, meaning the participants, researchers, and the trial sponsor are all unaware of treatment assignments. Blinding is essential to reduce bias.

📖 **Bias** is the unintentional influence of expectations or preconceived notions on the results. For example, if participants know they are receiving the experimental drug, they may interpret normal experiences (e.g., mild fatigue) as drug side effects, or they might report feeling better simply because they expect improvement. Similarly, researchers who know which participants are on the experimental drug may unconsciously interpret vague feedback like, "I feel slightly better," as a sign of improvement.

Blinding isn't always straightforward and can sometimes fail. For example, in trials testing weight-loss drugs, participants who start shedding pounds may suspect they are receiving the active treatment, potentially "**unblinding**" the trial. Also, if the active drug causes noticeable side effects, like severe nausea or diarrhea, participants or researchers may guess who is receiving the treatment.

In some cases, blinding may be impractical or unethical. For example, in surgical trials, the surgeons may know whether a full procedure or a sham was performed. In trials for physical or psychological therapy interventions, participants are often aware of the type of therapy they are receiving. In such situations, researchers may use strategies like centralized outcome assessment (where an independent third party evaluates results) or rely on objective **endpoints** (e.g., a biomarker) to minimize bias.

Blinding is a cornerstone of rigorous clinical trials. By reducing bias, it ensures that trial results are accurate, credible, and ultimately beneficial to patients. While challenges exist, careful planning and creative strategies can preserve the scientific integrity of the trial, even in complex scenarios.

Randomization: The Power of Chance

Imagine that, after a clinical trial is over and the data analysis is completed, the researchers conclude that the experimental drug successfully reduced the risk of stroke. However, upon closer examination, the patients who received the drug were, on average, fifteen years younger than those in the placebo group. Since stroke incidence increases with age, this imbalance would invalidate the findings, making it unclear whether the drug itself was effective or if the younger age of participants skewed the results.

To prevent such issues, trials use randomization, a process that assigns participants to treatment or placebo groups by chance rather than choice. Randomization helps to eliminate selection bias and ensures that the groups are comparable in terms of key factors like age, health status, and other variables that could influence the outcome. By balancing these factors between groups, randomization strengthens the reliability of the trial's conclusions.

Participants in a clinical trial are assigned to groups using a randomization process. However, it's not as simple as flipping a coin ("heads" for placebo, "tails" for the drug). While randomness is an essential component, the process is carefully structured to ensure balance and fairness across groups. If assignments were purely random, there's an exceedingly small but real possibility that all participants could end up in the same group, for example, everyone receiving the placebo. For instance, in a hypothetical trial of twenty participants, the probability that all twenty end up receiving the drug based on a coin toss would be about one in a million.

Despite such a minuscule possibility, one of the trial statisticians' jobs is to actively prevent these imbalances. One strategy is to use "block randomization," in which participants are grouped into small "blocks" to ensure an equal distribution between groups. For example, in a block of four participants, two might receive the drug and two the placebo, but their order is randomized (e.g., ABBA, BABA, or similar). This process is repeated for each new block, maintaining balance across the trial while preserving the element of chance.

While 1:1 randomization (equal chance of receiving placebo or drug) is the most common, some trials use asymmetric randomization ratios, such as 2:1 or 3:1. In these cases, participants have a higher likelihood of being assigned to the treatment group. For example, in a 2:1 randomization, two-thirds of participants receive the experimental drug, and only one-third receive the placebo. Asymmetric randomization is often used to increase participants' chances of receiving the active treatment, which can make the trial more appealing to potential volunteers, especially in cases of severe or life-threatening diseases.

Randomization ensures that any differences observed in the trial results can be attributed to the treatment itself, not to preexisting differences between the groups. By distributing participants with varying characteristics, such as age, sex, or disease severity, equally across the groups, researchers minimize bias and improve the reliability of the results.

For clinical trial participants, this means you cannot choose your group, and neither can the researchers. While this lack of control can feel frustrating, particularly for those hoping to receive the experimental drug, it is an essential part of ensuring the trial's integrity. Understanding the purpose and structure of randomization can help participants feel more at ease with this critical aspect of clinical trials.

Will You Ever Know to What Group You Were Assigned?

In a placebo-controlled trial, participants are deliberately kept unaware of whether they received the experimental drug, a placebo, or other control therapy to maintain the integrity of the study. Once the trial concludes, there is no legal requirement for researchers to inform participants about their group assignment.

However, in practice, many sponsors disclose this information at the end of the trial as a matter of transparency and to show appreciation for participants' contributions. Knowing whether they received the active treatment or a placebo can provide participants with closure and a better understanding of their experience in the trial.

Accepting or Rejecting Uncertainty

For some potential participants, the uncertainty inherent in clinical trials can be daunting. Yet, it's this very uncertainty that enables researchers to rigorously evaluate new therapies and ultimately bring effective treatments to patients worldwide. Understanding key elements like placebo, blinding, and randomization can empower you to make an informed decision about joining a trial.

While it may feel unsettling to participate in a trial without guarantees, your involvement contributes to the greater goal of advancing medical knowledge and improving outcomes for others. However, if the unknowns of a clinical trial feel overwhelming or incompatible with your comfort level, that's entirely valid. Clinical trials aren't for everyone, and choosing not to participate is a personal decision that deserves respect.

The Three Most Important Questions to Ask Yourself

Participating in a clinical trial involves weighing uncertainties and risks. In my experience, three key questions will help you decide if participating in a clinical trial could be the right choice for you:

1. Are you comfortable with the possibility of receiving an experimental drug that may or may not work, or that could have negative side effects?

2. Are you comfortable with the chance that you could receive a control therapy or placebo rather than the experimental treatment?

3. Are you comfortable with the uncertainty of not knowing whether you received the experimental drug or placebo during the trial?

If you answered *yes* to all three questions, clinical trials might align with your personality and goals. Despite the risks and uncertainties involved, you still find your participation valuable as it could contribute to life-changing advancements in medicine, potentially benefiting millions of people, even if they don't benefit you.

If you answered no to any of these questions, clinical trials might not be aligned with your personality and goals, and that's perfectly okay. Clinical trials are not for everyone. Discussing your concerns with your primary doctor, loved ones, or a clinical trial specialist can help you explore alternatives. Additionally, consider talking with a counselor or joining a support group if you feel conflicted. Making an informed decision is not just about your physical health but also your emotional readiness.

How to Discuss Clinical Trials with Your Doctor

If you're considering the possibility of participating in a clinical trial, your primary doctor could be a valuable ally in the decision-making process, even if they're not an expert on clinical trials. By approaching the conversation with clear goals and prepared questions, you could work together to explore whether a clinical trial is the right option for you or your loved one.

Step 1: Frame the Conversation

Start by explaining your interest in clinical trials and why you're thinking about them. This sets the tone for a productive discussion. For example:

- "I've been reading about clinical trials and wondering if they could be an option for my condition."
- "We're curious about experimental treatments and want to understand whether participating in a trial makes sense for us."

This approach signals that you're open to learning and making an informed decision together.

Step 2: Share Your Research

Doctors are very busy, and many are not actively involved in research or clinical trials. If you've found information about a specific trial or experimental treatment, share it during your visit. For example:

- "I came across a trial for my condition on ClinicalTrials.gov. Could we review it together?"
- "I heard about a new drug being tested. Do you think I might qualify for the trial?"

Provide your doctor with any relevant details you may have, such as trial location, **eligibility criteria**, and contact information. This gives them a starting point to offer guidance.

Step 3: Ask Targeted Questions

Your doctor might not have all the answers about a specific trial, but they can still help you assess whether it's worth pursuing. Consider asking questions like:

- "Do you think a clinical trial is a reasonable option for me? Why or why not?"
- "Do my medical records indicate that I might qualify for a trial?"
- "What aspects of my health or treatment history could affect my eligibility?"
- "Are there any risks I should be aware of before pursuing a trial?"

If your doctor is unfamiliar with clinical trials, ask if they can refer you to someone with more expertise, such as a clinical research coordinator or a specialist at a trial site. Patient advocacy groups often maintain up-to-date trial lists and can connect you with trial navigators who specialize in matching patients to suitable studies. Organizations like the National Comprehensive Cancer Network (NCCN) or disease-specific foundations can also provide tailored support. For instance, a parent of a child with a rare genetic disorder can turn to a patient advocacy group if their pediatrician is unfamiliar with trial options. These groups can help to identify suitable trials and navigate the application process, providing the support doctors sometimes can't offer.

Step 4: Discuss Logistics

If you're serious about participating in a trial, practical considerations come into play. Use this time to address logistical concerns:

- "Do you think I'll need additional tests or assessments to qualify for a trial?"
- "How would participating in a trial impact my current treatment plan?"
- "Could you coordinate with the trial team to share my medical history if I decide to apply?"
- "Will you remain involved in my medical care if I enroll in the trial?"

Having your doctor's support during the trial can provide continuity of care and reassurance.

⚠ Clinical trial participation is not a substitute for standard medical care. Clinical trial participants might still need to follow up with their primary doctor.

Step 5: Stay Proactive

Doctors may not always have time to explore all your options in-depth, so take the initiative to stay informed. Resources like ClinicalTrials.gov or patient advocacy groups can help you identify trials and provide additional guidance. If your doctor is hesitant about trials or dismisses the idea without explanation, politely advocate for yourself:

- "I understand that clinical trials aren't for everyone, but I'd like to explore all possibilities. Can we revisit this after I gather more information?"

Sometimes persistence is key to ensuring you explore every avenue.

The Role of Your Doctor in the Process

Even if your doctor isn't familiar with clinical trials, their insights into your medical history, current condition, and treatment goals can help you assess whether a trial aligns with your needs. They could help you to

- identify clinical trials for which you might qualify,
- review eligibility criteria and medical history,
- provide medical records or test results needed for trial enrollment, and
- offer guidance on balancing trial participation with existing care plans.

Your primary doctor might not have all the answers, but, still, a collaborative approach can make the process smoother and more empowering. Talking to your doctor about clinical trials is an important step in your journey.

By preparing in advance, asking thoughtful questions, and sharing your goals, you can ensure a productive conversation, even if your doctor isn't a clinical trials expert. Together, you can explore whether a trial is the right path forward, and if so, take steps to make informed and confident decisions.

Chapter 2 Highlights

- Participating in a clinical trial is a personal decision, offering hope while involving risks and uncertainties.
- Concepts like placebo, blinding, and randomization ensure that trials are scientifically rigorous but require participants to accept uncertainty.
- Potential risks include side effects, experimental treatments that may not work, and the time and logistical commitments involved.

- Clinical trial participation offers potential advantages such as access to cutting-edge therapies, high-quality medical care, and the opportunity to contribute to advancing medicine.
- Misconceptions about clinical trials, such as guaranteed treatment success or ongoing drug access after a trial, can lead to unrealistic expectations.
- Open communication with your doctor and self-reflection on your comfort with risks and uncertainties can help determine if clinical trials align with your goals.

Notes

1. Center for Information and Study on Clinical Research Participation (CISCRP), 2023, *Perceptions and Insights Study*, https://www.ciscrp.org/wp-content/uploads/2023/11/2023PI_Participation-Experiences.pdf (March 25, 2025).
2. Ibid.
3. W. Grant Thompson, MD, *The Placebo Effect and Health: Combining Science and Passionate Care* (New York: Prometheus Books), 2005.

3

Where to Start: Finding Clinical Trials

Participating in a clinical trial is not just about deciding if trials are right for you; it's about finding the proper trial for your needs and circumstances. Where do you begin? How do you sift through the options to find a trial that matches your unique condition, location, and preferences?

Finding a clinical trial can feel like searching for a needle in a haystack. This chapter is your roadmap, providing step-by-step guidance to searching and locating relevant trials. I will teach you how to use the most essential tool for finding clinical trials, ClinicalTrials.gov. I'll also discuss strategies for improving your search results, interpreting trial information, and discovering additional resources to help streamline your search.

While searching for a clinical trial is never easy, this chapter aims to equip you with the knowledge and resources to make it as efficient and targeted as possible, ensuring you can identify trials that meet your needs and align with your goals.

How to Search for Clinical Trials

Searching for a clinical trial isn't as simple as typing your condition into a search engine. It can be an overwhelming and frustrating experience, more so if you or your loved one is suffering from a rapidly progressive disease, and time and hope are running short.

🔍 When Lucas faced a recurrence of an aggressive cancer, his wife immediately contacted his oncologist at a leading medical institution. The response, though polite, was devastating. There were no effective therapies available for his advanced disease, and the only chemotherapy option offered was limited to "palliative and symptomatic" care, unlikely to change Lucas's already grim prognosis.

Undeterred, Lucas's wife asked about clinical trials. The oncologist's reply was discouraging: "Oh, we can discuss clinical trials, but at a later date." For someone confronting an aggressive cancer, "later" wasn't an option. Driven by urgency, Lucas and his wife turned to their personal networks and reached out to online physician communities and colleagues across the country. Despite their good intentions, useful recommendations were hard to come by. Well-meaning responses from physicians often consisted of general advice like, "Try contacting a large research center," or vague suggestions to "check ClinicalTrials.gov." Even when other doctors searched the database using Lucas's clinical details, the results varied significantly; no two searches surfaced the same trial options.

This inconsistency highlights one of the major challenges in finding clinical trials: the process is neither straightforward nor user friendly. Patients and caregivers often find themselves navigating a labyrinth of complex medical terminology, unclear eligibility criteria, and incomplete information, all while racing against time. Reaching out to your network or posting in online forums might provide a starting point, but these efforts are seldom fruitful.

It's crucial to approach the search for clinical trials with both preparation and persistence. The process requires focus, organization, and an understanding of the resources available to you. It will involve some trial (no pun intended!) and error. But with the right approach, you can uncover opportunities that could transform your treatment journey. The following will help you organize your research and understand how to use the resources so you can find proper clinical trials.

Start with a Clear Understanding of Your Condition

Before diving into clinical trial databases, take the time to understand the nuances of your diagnosis. Knowing these details can refine your search and help you identify trials that are most relevant to your situation.

1. What is the medical term for your condition? Many diseases have both common and scientific names. For instance, ALS might be referred to as "Lou Gehring disease," "amyotrophic lateral sclerosis," or "motor neuron disease." Using the proper terminology in your search (and expanding the search to include the different terms used for your condition) can help yield more results, especially in databases like ClinicalTrials.gov.

2. If you have a cancer diagnosis, what is the histological type? General terms like "lung cancer" or "skin cancer" are often too broad to be helpful when searching for clinical trials. Knowing the histological type of your cancer is essential, as it provides specific details about the cancer's cellular characteristics, which are typically determined through a biopsy. For example, skin cancer could be melanoma, basal cell carcinoma, or

adenocarcinoma, among other rarer types. This specificity is crucial because clinical trials are often designed for particular histological subtypes.

3. Are there genetic variants of your disease? Some conditions have subtypes that influence treatment options and trial eligibility. For instance, some forms of ALS are linked to genetic mutations, like SOD1 or C9orf72. Similarly, some forms of Parkinson's disease are linked to genetic mutations in LRRK2 or GBA. Trials targeting these mutations might exclude patients without them. Many cancers are classified by genetic mutations (e.g., HER2-positive breast cancer or EGFR-mutated lung cancer). Many trials for targeted therapies often require patients to have these specific mutations. Knowing your subtype can save time and help you zero in on trials designed for your condition.

4. What is the stage of your disease? The disease stage often determines trial eligibility. Researchers use standardized scales to classify stages. For cancer, staging often includes factors like tumor size, lymph node involvement, and metastasis (e.g., Stage I to IV). For neurological diseases like Parkinson's, scales like the Hoehn and Yahr staging help determine severity. Many cancer trials use functional scales, such as the Karnofsky Performance Status or the ECOG Performance Status, to measure patients' ability to perform daily activities. Understanding your disease stage and how it aligns with a trial's criteria is important for determining eligibility.

5. Is your condition progressive, stable, or acute? Understanding the nature of your condition and whether it is progressive, stable, or acute can help you set realistic expectations for clinical trial goals. Progressive conditions, such as Alzheimer's

disease, most cancers, or Parkinson's disease, worsen over time. Clinical trials for progressive diseases often aim to slow or halt the progression of the condition, though some trials may focus on improving specific bothersome symptoms (e.g., reducing hallucinations in Parkinson's disease or ameliorating pain in cancer patients). Stable, nonprogressive conditions, like chronic migraine or, very slowly progressive, such as osteoarthritis, typically have clinical trials that focus on symptom management and improving quality of life. Acute conditions, such as bacterial infections or appendicitis, are short-term issues where trials often aim to achieve resolution of the problem or prevent complications. Recognizing whether your condition is progressive, stable, or acute allows you to better understand what a trial aims to accomplish and evaluate whether those goals align with your treatment priorities.

6   What are the available, approved treatments for your condition? Understanding the existing treatment landscape is critical when considering a trial. For instance, if you're considering a trial for metastatic breast cancer, compare the experimental therapy's goals to those of available options like hormone therapies or immunotherapy. If the experimental treatment aims to achieve the same outcome as an approved therapy (e.g., symptom management), ask yourself and your doctor whether the potential benefits of participating in the trial outweigh the risks and uncertainties. Alternatively, some trials could allow you to receive the experimental drug on top of any standard-of-care treatment. Knowing what's already available empowers you to assess whether a trial is worth pursuing and whether it offers something novel or superior.

Asking these questions upfront helps you focus your search and avoid wasting time on trials for which you're unlikely to qualify. It also provides a structured approach for discussing your options with your healthcare provider and the clinical trial team. As the old slogan from a clothing store once said, "An educated consumer is our best customer." The same applies to clinical trials; a well-informed participant is better positioned to find studies that truly align with their medical needs and personal priorities.

A Step-by-Step Guide to Using ClinicalTrials.gov

ClinicalTrials.gov is the most comprehensive public registry of clinical trials worldwide. Established in 2000 and managed by the US National Library of Medicine (NLM) and the National Institutes of Health (NIH), it provides detailed information on thousands of trials conducted in the United States and internationally.

ClinicalTrials.gov provides a wealth of information, including:

- Trial Locations: Details about where trials are being conducted.
- Eligibility Criteria: Requirements for participation in the trial, such as age, sex, disease stage, or prior treatments.
- Trial Status: Whether the trial is recruiting, completed, or not yet open for enrollment.
- Study Details: Information on the sponsor, objectives, and study design.
- Contact Information: Points of contact for each trial.

This invaluable resource is freely accessible online, but its vast scope and complexity can make it daunting for first-time users.

In this section, I'll guide you through navigating ClinicalTrials.gov effectively, helping you find the trials most relevant to your needs.

Step 1: Start Your Search

Begin by visiting ClinicalTrials.gov. You'll find a search bar on the homepage labeled "Find a Study."

At first glance, it might seem straightforward, so let's dive in and search for clinical trials. Suppose you're looking for trials related to Parkinson's disease. In the "Condition/Disease" field, type "Parkinson's disease" and select the auto-populated option "Parkinson Disease." Then, hit "Search." In my search, this yielded 4,041 studies!

However, this list includes a mix of interventional clinical trials and observational (noninterventional) studies.

📖 **Interventional trials** actively test treatments or procedures to evaluate their effect, such as testing a new drug for Alzheimer's. As discussed in Chapter 1, interventions can be pharmacological and non-pharmacological.

📖 **Observational (noninterventional) studies**, in contrast, gather data without altering participants' care or administering experimental treatments, like tracking Parkinson's patients' walking patterns to find early markers of disease progression.

⚠ Understanding the difference between interventional and observational studies is key to narrowing your search. For example, if you're looking for clinical trials that provide access to experimental therapies, ensure that your results are filtered to interventional studies only. Observational studies might still be of interest if you're interested in contributing data to help future treatments.

Additionally, ClinicalTrials.gov covers not only active, recruiting studies but also completed trials, some of which concluded decades ago. While the volume of results might feel overwhelming, don't worry, we can refine the results to make them more relevant.

Step 2: Refine Your Search Results

With potentially hundreds of results, refining your search is crucial. Use the filters on the left-hand side to narrow the options as much as possible:

- Recruitment status: Select "Recruiting" to focus on trials actively seeking participants.
- Location: Filter by country, state, or city to find trials near you.
- Age range: Select the age you or your loved one belong to.
- Phase: Choose the trial phase (or phases) based on your preferences (e.g., Phase 1, 2, or 3).
- Study Type: Make sure you opt for interventional studies if you're seeking treatment trials (remember, this will include pharmacological and non-pharmacological interventions).

In the example above, to narrow my search, I filtered for interventional Phase 1, Phase 2, and Phase 3 trials that are actively "Recruiting" older adults (sixty-five-plus) in California. This reduced the results to fourteen studies, a much more manageable number.

Among these fourteen studies, several studied non-pharmacological interventions (such as gamification and transcranial magnetic stimulation) or were drug-repurposing trials (e.g., adrenergic blockers). However, only four or five trials investigated experimental therapies to slow or halt Parkinson's disease progression. These included experimental treatments such as antibodies, oral medications, gene therapy, and dopaminergic cell transplantation. These clinical trials, testing experimental drugs often identified by code names like BIIB122 or UCB022 (indicating sponsorship by pharmaceutical companies), could be appealing options for patients interested in exploring cutting-edge treatments for Parkinson's disease.

If you're open to traveling for clinical trials, you can broaden your search. For example, instead of limiting the location to California, simply enter "USA" in the search field. This will increase the number of available trials and give you many more options.

💡 Pro Tip: Once you find a clinical trial that interests you, be sure to note down (or copy and paste to a document or spreadsheet) its NCT number (e.g., NCT06055985), the one that shows up above or below the trial's name. This unique ID number will make it much easier to find the trial again on ClinicalTrials.gov. Simply enter the NCT number in the "Other terms" field on the homepage, and the trial will appear immediately, saving you time and effort.

Step 3: Understand the Study Details

Click on a study title to view its detailed record. Here's what to focus on:

1 Phase: The trial phase is listed on the right side of the record, along with other key details such as the study's start date, estimated completion date, and the number of participants to be enrolled. For instance, clinical trial NCT06055985 is a Phase 2 trial. As discussed in previous chapters, earlier-phase trials (e.g., Phase 1 or 2) involve more experimental drugs with higher levels of uncertainty. If you're risk-averse or prefer a higher likelihood of success, consider looking at Phase 3 studies, where the drug has already shown promising results in earlier phases.

⚠ Just because a drug is being tested in a Phase 3 clinical trial, that doesn't necessarily mean the Phase 2 trial was positive. Sometimes, for complex reasons, biotech and pharmaceutical companies move forward with Phase 3 trials despite mixed or disappointing Phase 2 data.

🔍 One example is verdiperstat, an experimental drug initially developed by AstraZeneca for multiple system atrophy (MSA), a rare and rapidly progressive parkinsonian disorder. In Phase 2 trials, verdiperstat failed to demonstrate sufficient clinical benefit and showed no significant biological effect in the brain, as assessed by specialized imaging studies. AstraZeneca subsequently sold the drug to Biohaven Pharmaceuticals. Despite the lackluster Phase 2 results, Biohaven decided to move forward with a Phase 3 trial. This placebo-controlled study enrolled 336 participants but ultimately failed to show efficacy in slowing disease progression. Following these disappointing outcomes, the program was discontinued. This case highlights the significant risks of advancing a drug to Phase 3 without robust evidence of efficacy and safety from earlier studies.

2. Study Overview and Brief Summary: This section outlines the trial's primary objective. It may be written in technical terms but provides essential information. For example, NCT06055985 states: "To demonstrate the superiority of UCB022 as an adjunctive treatment to standard-of-care over placebo with regards to motor fluctuations in participants with advanced Parkinson's disease." By reading carefully, you can glean that this trial is testing whether the drug UCB022 improves motor fluctuations when added to standard Parkinson's medications. In other words, the study aims to improve symptoms, not to slow the disease progression. Also, the study is recruiting participants with advanced Parkinson's disease, as these are the ones who likely suffer from motor fluctuations and are already receiving standard-of-care medications. It's important to assess whether these conditions align with your own or your loved one's situation.

💡 Pro Tip: The "Study Overview" section in ClinicalTrials.gov often specifies the route of administration for the experimental drug; whether it's taken orally (as a capsule or tablet), intravenously (via infusion or injection), subcutaneously (under the skin), or intrathecally (through a lumbar puncture or spinal tap). This information is crucial in selecting a trial that aligns with your circumstances and comfort levels. For example, if you experience swallowing difficulties, an oral medication might not be the best option. Similarly, intrathecal administration requires spinal taps, which some participants may find daunting. Pay close attention to this section to avoid surprises.

3. Contacts and Locations: This section includes contact details and participating study sites. Sometimes individual site emails and phone numbers are listed, enabling potential participants to reach out to research sites. In other cases, only a general contact from the sponsor (e.g., the pharmaceutical company) is provided.

4. Participation Criteria and Eligibility: This section specifies who can participate. Read the Inclusion Criteria (who can join) and Exclusion Criteria (who cannot join) carefully. For example, in NCT06055985, participants must be aged thirty-five to sixty-five, have a Parkinson's diagnosis for at least five years, and be at a Hoehn and Yahr stage of three or less. Additionally, the trial excludes individuals with other serious neurological or medical conditions. These criteria are nonnegotiable and ensure the safety and consistency of the trial (more on clinical trial eligibility in the next section).

5. What Is the Study Measuring? This section describes the primary outcomes or scales the trial will use to determine success. For instance, you might see terms like "motor function," "disease progression," or "quality of life."

💡 Pro Tip: Look for the "Time Frame" section, which indicates how long participants will be required to be part of the study. In NCT06055985, the longest time frame listed is Week 12, suggesting that participants will need to commit to the trial for at least three months, and perhaps slightly longer.

Feeling overwhelmed at this point? Don't worry, it's perfectly normal. ClinicalTrials.gov is far from user friendly and is packed with technical jargon that can be difficult to digest, especially for first-time users. Terms like "**futility**," "**open-label**," "**crossover design**," or "**delayed-start**" might be confusing. Use the glossary provided on the site (https://clinicaltrials.gov/study-basics/glossary) or take a look at the glossary section at the end of this book for clarification.

It's okay if you need to read through the trial details multiple times to extract the most relevant information (trust me, even I have to do this!).

💡 Pro Tip: To help you stay organized and make the process more manageable make sure you track your trials. You can create a spreadsheet or document to organize the clinical trials that catch your interest. Include columns for key details like the NCT number, drug name, sponsor, phase, study goal, inclusion criteria, exclusion criteria, duration, and contact information. I provide more details on how to create this spreadsheet in Chapter 4. Consolidating this information in one place will make it much easier to compare your options and manage your search.

Take it step by step and remember that feeling a bit lost can be part of the process. With patience and a system to keep you organized, you'll be better equipped to navigate the database and identify trials that may be a good fit for you.

ClinicalTrials.gov is a powerful tool, but it's not perfect. If you find the interface cumbersome or your results unclear, don't despair; it may take some time to get used to it. If you still have trouble finding results, make sure you check out the "Other Resources and Websites for Finding Trials" section later in this chapter.

Can Artificial Intelligence Chatbots Help to Find Clinical Trials?

Artificial intelligence (AI) has transformed countless aspects of daily life, from generating emails and tackling complex problems to enhancing creative pursuits. Its influence on healthcare has the potential to be revolutionary.

AI-powered tools such as chatbots, predictive algorithms, and diagnostic systems are poised to reshape medical practice.[1] Some experts even suggest that medical specialties like radiology or pathology might one day be fully automated, given AI's capabilities for pattern recognition and data analysis.

With AI's increasing role in healthcare, it's reasonable to ask: Could AI help patients find the perfect clinical trial? To explore this question, I decided to test ChatGPT (specifically the GPT-4-turbo model) by prompting a real-world scenario:

User: "Assume the role of an expert clinical trials navigator. You are familiar with the databases that list active clinical trials. I am a caregiver who is interested in finding a Phase 2 clinical trial that is currently recruiting pediatric patients (my child is 12 years old) with a diagnosis of sarcoma of the bone, in an early stage of the disease, with no metastasis. Can you give me a list of suitable trials?"

ChatGPT: *"It looks like I wasn't able to access clinical trial databases directly, but you can search for suitable trials using*

ClinicalTrials.gov, which is the most comprehensive database for active clinical trials. Here's how you can do it:

Step-by-Step Guide to Finding a Suitable Trial:

- Go to ClinicalTrials.gov
- Enter Search Terms:
    - Condition: "Bone sarcoma" or a more specific type like "Osteosarcoma" or "Ewing Sarcoma"
    - Other Keywords: "pediatric" or "child" (to refine for pediatric patients)
    - Recruitment Status: Select "Recruiting" and "Not Yet Recruiting"
    - Phase: Select "Phase 2"
    - Age Criteria: Enter your child's age (12 years old)
    - Refine by Location: If you have a preference for specific countries or regions, use the filters.
- Review Trial Details: Click on individual trials to check inclusion/exclusion criteria, treatment details, and contact information.

Would you like me to help interpret any trial details or guide you in reaching out to trial sites? Let me know how I can assist further!"

So, not very useful, as ChatGPT can't directly search trial databases like ClinicalTrials.gov, at least not by the time this book was printed (although this could change in the near future as technology advances). This means that you still must do the work of searching ClinicalTrials.gov by yourself.

There are other, more specialized tools. For instance, the Dana-Farber Cancer Institute has developed an AI-based MatchMiner platform,[2] and the NIH developed an AI-based chatbot called TrialGPT.[3] Unfortunately, none of these are freely available to the public, at least in user-friendly interfaces (you might be able to use TrialGPT if you are an expert in coding and large language processing tools, though).

So, while AI-based chatbots have the potential to help people find suitable clinical trials, the technology is still in its infancy.

Other Resources and Websites for Finding Trials

While ClinicalTrials.gov remains the gold standard for locating clinical trials, it's not the only resource available. Many other platforms and organizations offer tools to help you navigate this complex process, each with unique strengths and limitations. Here's an overview of some of the most useful resources.

International Clinical Trial Registries

ClinicalTrials.gov focuses on US-based studies, although it also includes many international studies. There are also numerous international databases and registries listing clinical trials conducted outside of the United States; some are listed in Table 3.1.

These resources could be useful if you are willing and able to seek treatment options in other countries. Like ClinicalTrials.gov, most of these registries include trial information, including eligibility criteria, study locations, and contact details, helping patients and clinicians explore treatment options beyond their home countries.

Table 3.1 Clinical Trial Registries

Clinical Trial Registry	Geography of Interest	Website
ClinicalTrials.gov	USA and global	https://clinicaltrials.gov
Australian New Zealand Clinical Trials Registry (ANZCTR)	Australia and New Zealand	https://www.anzctr.org.au
Health Canada Clinical Trials Database	Canada	https://health-products.canada.ca/ctdb-bdec/?lang=eng
Brazilian Clinical Trials Registry (ReBec)	Brazil	https://ensaiosclinicos.gov.br
Chinese Clinical Trial Registry (ChiCTR)	China	https://www.chictr.org.cn
International Traditional Chinese Medicine Clinical Trial Registry (ITMCTR)	China	http://itmctr.ccebtcm.org.cn/en-US
Clinical Research Information Service (CRiS), Republic of Korea	Republic of Korea (South Korea)	https://cris.nih.go.kr/cris/info/introduce.do?search_lang=E&lang=E
Clinical Trials Registry—India (CTRI)	India	https://ctri.nic.in/Clinicaltrials/login.php
Clinical Research Site—MyTrial	Israel	https://my.health.gov.il/CliniTrials/Pages/Home.aspx
Cuban Public Registry of Clinical Trials (RPCEC)	Cuba	https://rpcec.sld.cu/en
EU Clinical Trials Register (EU-CTR)	European Union	https://euclinicaltrials.eu/search-for-clinical-trials/trial-map/?lang=en
Iranian Registry of Clinical Trials (IRCT)	Iran	https://www.irct.ir

Clinical Trial Registry	Geography of Interest	Website
Japan Registry of Clinical Trials (jRCT)	Japan	https://jrct.niph.go.jp
Lebanese Clinical Trials Registry (LBCTR)	Lebanon	https://lbctr.moph.gov.lb
Thai Clinical Trials Registry (TCTR)	Thailand	https://thaiclinicaltrials.org
Pan African Clinical Trial Registry (PACTR)	Africa	https://pactr.samrc.ac.za
Peruvian Clinical Trial Registry (REPEC)	Peru	https://ensayosclinicos-repec.ins.gob.pe/en/
Sri Lanka Clinical Trials Registry (SLCTR)	Sri Lanka	https://www.slctr.lk

⚠ While international registries could provide additional resources, most clinical trials, including those conducted outside the United States, are already listed on ClinicalTrials.gov. As a result, these international registries may not necessarily help you discover new trials.

If you do find a promising trial in another country, be aware of potential logistical and regulatory challenges, such as:

- visa and immigration requirements for medical stays;
- health insurance coverage; some countries require proof of coverage for medical care;
- travel and accommodation logistics, especially for long-term participation; and
- language barriers that could hinder communication with the clinical trial team.

Carefully evaluating these factors can help you determine whether a trial abroad is a viable option.

National Cancer Institute (NCI)

The National Cancer Institute (NCI), a branch of the NIH dedicated to cancer research, provides its own clinical trial search tool at https://www.cancer.gov/research/participate/clinical-trials-search. This registry is tailored specifically to NCI-funded trials. However, keep in mind that all these trials are also listed on ClinicalTrials.gov, so using the NCI's database might result in duplicate information. Nonetheless, its streamlined focus on cancer trials could make it a helpful resource for patients seeking oncology trials.

Patient Advocacy Groups and Disease-Specific Organizations

Organizations dedicated to specific diseases or conditions often maintain their own trial databases or provide guidance tailored to their patient communities. These groups can be a treasure trove of information, offering personalized support and resources. When using resources like patient advocacy groups, ensure that they align with your condition's specific needs. Some resources cater primarily to certain diseases.

For example, the Michael J. Fox Foundation for Parkinson's Research site includes the Fox Trial Finder (https://www.michaeljfox.org/trial-finder), an efficient, user-friendly, free trial finder tool, specifically for Parkinson's disease, which includes filters for location, trial type, and participation criteria.

Disease-specific organizations can also be excellent resources for finding clinical trial listings. For instance, Breast Cancer Trials offers free, tailored search engines specifically designed for breast cancer patients (https://www.breastcancertrials.org/BCTIncludes/index.html). These tools cater to different stages of the disease; one focuses on early-stage breast cancer (Stages 0-III), while another is dedicated to metastatic breast cancer (Stage IV). By incorporating detailed patient data, such as genetic mutations, histological cancer type, and other specific factors, these search engines make the process of identifying relevant trials more precise and personalized.

Rare disease foundations frequently have their clinical trial listings. For instance, the Cystic Fibrosis Foundation provides an up-to-date registry of clinical trials for patients with cystic fibrosis (https://apps.cff.org/trials/finder). These organizations understand the nuances of specific diseases and often include resources like patient navigators, who can help you through the process of finding and enrolling in trials.

Hospital and Research Center Websites

Large hospitals and academic research centers often conduct clinical trials and list them on their websites. If you are already receiving care at a specific institution, their website is an excellent starting point for finding trials. Some examples are:

- Memorial Sloan Kettering Cancer Center (New York, NY): Provides a searchable list of ongoing cancer clinical trials: https://www.mskcc.org/cancer-care/clinical-trials.

- New York University Langone Health (New York, NY): Features a comprehensive database on interventional and noninterventional studies for a variety of diseases: https://clinicaltrials.med.nyu.edu.

- MD Anderson Cancer Center (Houston, TX): Lists cancer trials, searchable by type and stage: (https://www.mdanderson.org/patients-family/diagnosis-treatment/clinical-trials.html).

- Bascom Palmer Eye Institute, University of Miami (Miami, FL): Renowned as one of the leading research institutions in ophthalmology, Bascom Palmer participates in numerous clinical trials, many of which are multicenter studies: https://umiamihealth.org/bascom-palmer-eye-institute/clinical-trials.
- Mayo Clinic (multiple locations): Features a comprehensive database of trials conducted at its facilities, including both interventional and observational studies: (https://www.mayo.edu/research/clinical-trials).

Many other academic medical centers have similar sites. Make sure you check them out, particularly if you live nearby or if you are already a patient in their network. These websites are often more detailed about the specific logistics of the trials conducted at that institution, including contact information for local coordinators.

Pharmaceutical Company Websites

Pharmaceutical companies developing new therapies often maintain their own clinical trial portals. These can be especially useful if you're looking for trials involving a specific experimental drug. For example:

- Pfizer Clinical Trials: https://www.pfizerclinicaltrials.com
- Novartis Clinical Trials: https://www.novartis.com/clinicaltrials
- Roche Clinical Trials: https://forpatients.roche.com
- Johnson & Johnson: https://clinicaltrials.jnj.com/en

Other pharmaceutical companies should have similar listings. If you know the name of a specific drug or are interested in a company's pipeline, these websites can provide detailed, up-to-date trial information.

Social Media and Online Communities

While not a primary source for finding trials, social media platforms and online patient communities could sometimes point you in the right direction. Some patients and caregivers might share their experiences with trials. Commonly used platforms include Facebook Groups, Reddit, Smart Patients (an online community where patients discuss clinical trials and treatments), or HealthUnlocked (a forum with groups focused on various conditions, where clinical trial-related discussions are common). These platforms could offer peer support and firsthand accounts of trial participation, which could help you gauge what to expect.

Trial-Matching Platforms

Trial-matching platforms act as third-party intermediaries, connecting patients with ongoing clinical trials. They are neither trial sponsors nor clinical research sites but serve as a bridge to help patients navigate the often-complicated landscape of clinical trials. These platforms use a variety of tools, including AI (at least that's what they claim), to match patients based on their medical profiles, conditions, and other relevant factors.

These platforms typically require patients to provide personal information, including medical records, genetic data, or demographic details, which can raise privacy concerns. Their business models vary, some are for-profit entities supported by fees from sponsors, while others operate as nonprofits offering free services. Here are four examples.

- ResearchMatch: This platform allows prospective study volunteers to enter their data, joining a "volunteer pool." They then receive email notifications about relevant studies.

ResearchMatch is free to use for everyone and includes a range of noninterventional studies.

- Antidote: Antidote offers a user-friendly questionnaire to match patients with clinical trials. To view results, users must provide an email address and accept the platform's terms of use and privacy policy. As a for-profit organization, Antidote receives payment from sponsors and research organizations for recruitment services, with no cost to patients.

- LealHealth (formerly TrialJectory): LealHealth, which focuses on oncology, claims to use AI to analyze patients' medical records and recommend appropriate clinical trials. To access their services, patients must upload a copy of their medical records and accept the platform's privacy policy and terms of use. LealHealth is a for-profit organization, funded by sponsors and research organizations for recruitment services, with no costs to patients.

- CenterWatch: CenterWatch provides a comprehensive database of clinical trials along with educational resources. The platform offers both free access for patients seeking trial information and premium, subscription-based services for professionals with advanced tools.

There are many other matching services out there. While these tools aim to make trial searching more accessible, their actual effectiveness can vary. On the one hand, they can simplify searches by filtering irrelevant trials and make personalized recommendations. On the other hand, these platforms frequently miss trials due to incomplete or outdated information. They claim to solve all trial-matching challenges, but they may fall short, and the AI methods they claim to use, and matching criteria are often unclear. Moreover, there are privacy concerns, as patients must share sensitive data, raising questions about data security and usage, and these platforms may retain your data indefinitely even if their services are not used. In the for-profit platforms that are funded by sponsors, it is unclear if they would prioritize specific trials over others, compromising objectivity.

If you still want to use one of these platforms, look for clear explanations of their data sources, matching methods, and funding; research reviews or endorsements from trusted organizations; and ensure they have robust data security measures and clear policies on data retention.

⚠ Beware of red flags when dealing with trial-matching platforms. No platform can guarantee trial acceptance. This is something that only an investigator at the research site can determine. Beware of services that use emotional appeals or urgency to push for enrollment. Avoid platforms that provide vague or generic trial descriptions.

In my opinion, there are better alternatives to the use of these platforms. Free and reputable options, such as ClinicalTrials.gov or hospital trial registries, often provide comprehensive trial listings without the potential concerns associated with third-party platforms. Additionally, disease-specific advocacy groups or nonprofit trial-matching services may offer free personalized assistance. Your time, money, and health are too valuable to waste on services that may not deliver.

When No Trials Are Available

Despite a strong commitment to participating in clinical trials, you may find that none are currently available for your specific disease, stage, or location. In fact, a little over half of cancer patients face this reality.[4]

Reaching a dead end in your search for clinical trials can feel discouraging, but it doesn't necessarily mean all options are exhausted. Alternative pathways may still provide access to experimental treatments or emerging therapies. These routes often require persistence, extensive paperwork, and proactive advocacy on your part, but they can offer hope in otherwise difficult circumstances.

This section delves into key alternatives, including expanded access programs, right-to-try laws, and the possibility of pursuing personalized genetic medicine approaches, such as therapies tailored specifically to your or your loved one's condition.

Each option has unique requirements, potential benefits, and limitations, which we'll break down to help you navigate this complex landscape effectively. With determination and knowledge, even the absence of existing trials doesn't have to mean the absence of options.

The FDA Expanded Access Program

The FDA's **Expanded Access Program** (EAP), often referred to as "compassionate use" or "single patient exception," allows patients with serious or life-threatening conditions to access investigational treatments outside of clinical trials; patients must meet specific criteria. Specifically, patients must:

- have a serious or life-threatening condition,
- have exhausted all approved treatment options, and
- be unable to enroll in an appropriate clinical trial (or no clinical trials are available).

While this program provides access to investigational treatments, it does not guarantee success or eliminate risks. Patients should understand that these treatments are still under investigation and may not work as intended. The process involves several steps:

1. Determine Eligibility: Patients must meet the criteria for expanded access, including the inability to enroll in an active clinical trial.
2. Physician Request: The treating physician must contact the drug manufacturer to request access to the investigational therapy (most pharmaceutical companies have specific web pages to initiate the process).
3. Pharmaceutical Company Agreement: The company must agree to provide the drug.

⚠ Pharmaceutical and biotechnology companies are not legally required to provide access to an investigational drug through an EAP, nor are they obligated to offer it free of charge. Availability depends on company policies, drug supply, regulatory approvals, and other factors.

4. Submit to FDA: The physician submits an **Investigational New Drug (IND) application** to the FDA, including a treatment plan and patient history. For emergencies, this process can be expedited and approved within hours.
5. IRB Review: A local IRB reviews and approves the request to ensure that the treatment aligns with ethical guidelines.
6. Begin Treatment: Once all approvals are secured, the patient can start receiving the treatment under the physician's supervision.

The advantages of the EAP are that it ensures safety and ethical standards as it requires both FDA and IRB approval. Moreover, physicians must report treatment outcomes to the FDA, contributing to medical knowledge.

Potential disadvantages are that drug companies are not required to provide the treatment and may decline due to limited supply or concerns about the benefit-risk assessment. As with any experimental therapy, the treatment may not work and could pose unforeseen risks.

⚠ The FDA does not charge a fee for an EAP application. However, patients (or their insurance) may need to cover significant costs, including the experimental drug itself, related medical care, and administrative expenses. It's essential to clarify in advance whether these costs will be covered by the pharmaceutical company, the treating hospital, or the patient's insurance. Some drug manufacturers offer patient assistance programs to help offset some expenses, and many will provide the experimental drug at no cost.

⚠ Before pursuing an EAP, consider all available options. If a clinical trial is an option, it is crucial to prioritize trial participation over an EAP. Applying for an EAP to avoid the possibility of receiving a placebo in a clinical trial is unethical. It can undermine the integrity of ongoing research and fairness to other trial participants and is unlikely to be approved by the pharmaceutical company sponsoring the drug. Furthermore, clinical trials often provide advantages that EAPs do not, such as more rigorous monitoring, access to the experimental drug at no cost, and, in some cases, financial compensation for participation-related expenses. These benefits make clinical trials a more structured and reliable pathway for patients whenever available. EAPs are only considered when no trials are accessible or suitable, and patients must have exhausted all other therapeutic and investigational options before applying.

The "Right-to-Try" Laws: A Last Resort for Patients

In 2018, President Trump signed the "Right-to-Try Act" law, creating another potential pathway for terminally ill patients to access experimental therapies outside of clinical trials. Designed as a last resort for individuals with no other treatment options, the law provides an alternative to the FDA's EAP. While the Right-to-Try Act may sound promising, it is essential to understand its limitations and the rights it confers.

The Right-to-Try Act allows eligible patients to request access to investigational drugs that have passed Phase 1 clinical trials but have not yet been approved by the FDA. The law aims to bypass some of the bureaucratic hurdles associated with the FDA's EAP by eliminating the need for FDA approval. The intent is to give patients faster access to potentially lifesaving treatments. To qualify under this law:

1 Patients must have a life-threatening disease or condition and have exhausted all approved treatment options.

2 Drugs must have completed a Phase 1 clinical trial, and not yet be FDA approved for widespread use.

3 Physicians must certify that the patient meets eligibility criteria and discuss the potential risks involved.

Despite its name, the Right-to-Try Act does not compel any party to act, rendering it more symbolic than actionable in many cases.

⚠ Like the FDA's EAP, drug manufacturers are not required to provide the requested treatment as part of the Right-to-Try. They may decline due to production limitations, safety concerns, or reluctance to risk negative outcomes that could impact a future FDA approval of the drug. Also, like the EAP, the law does not require insurance companies, Medicare, or Medicaid to cover the costs associated with the investigational drug or related medical care. This leaves patients potentially facing steep out-of-pocket expenses.

⚠ Unlike the FDA's EAP, which requires data collection and oversight, the Right-to-Try Act does not mandate any reporting or monitoring. This lack of regulatory scrutiny may raise safety concerns.

In fact, since its passage, the Right-to-Try Act has had a minimal impact. Very few patients have successfully obtained experimental treatments under this law, and critics argue that the existing FDA EAP, while requiring more paperwork, is the more viable and practical pathway for most patients. Pharmaceutical companies often prefer the FDA's oversight and the liability protections it provides.

If you are considering the Right-to-Try Act as an option, follow these steps:

1. Consult your physician: Discuss whether this pathway aligns with your condition and treatment goals.
2. Contact the drug manufacturer: Ask if they are willing to provide the investigational treatment under the Right-to-Try Act.
3. Understand the financial implications: Be prepared for potentially high costs, as you will likely bear the financial burden of the drug and associated care.

While the Right-to-Try Act offers a theoretical option for terminally ill patients seeking experimental therapies, it does not solve many of the practical challenges inherent in accessing these treatments. When possible, patients should consider the FDA's EAP as a better alternative.

Bespoke Therapies

Advances in personalized medicine have opened a new frontier, offering hope even in the most challenging disorders, particularly for genetically defined diseases caused by rare mutations. Mila Makovec, a young girl diagnosed with an ultra-rare form of Batten disease, a pediatric genetic neurodegenerative disorder caused by a mutation in the CLN7 gene, exemplifies this possibility.

Where to Start

🔍 Mila's story began when she started showing symptoms of neurodegeneration at the age of three. By the time she was six, her condition had progressed rapidly, causing blindness, difficulty walking, and life-threatening seizures. Traditional treatment options were nonexistent, and no clinical trials were available for her rare mutation. Her mother, determined to find answers, sought help from researchers specializing in rare diseases. In a groundbreaking effort, a team led by Dr. Timothy Yu at Boston Children's Hospital developed milasen, a customized antisense oligonucleotide specifically designed to address Mila's unique genetic mutation. Remarkably, the entire process, from identifying the mutation to creating and administering the therapy, was completed in just over a year. Milasen was not a commercial drug and was created exclusively for Mila. It won't work in other patients unless they have the same mutation as Mila. It required exceptional collaboration among scientists, regulatory agencies, and Mila's family. While the therapy could not cure her disease, it slowed her condition's progression and significantly improved her quality of life for a time.

Mila's case highlights an important point: even when no clinical trials are available, there may still be avenues for developing highly individualized treatments for genetic disorders. This path, however, is not without challenges. Personalized therapies often require significant time, funding, and FDA oversight. They are also typically available only at highly specialized research centers with expertise in rare genetic diseases. If you or your loved one is facing a similar situation, consider reaching out to research institutions, advocacy groups, or specialists in your condition. Mila's story demonstrates that even in the absence of conventional trials, innovation and determination can sometimes create new possibilities.

One leading organization in this area is the n-Lorem Foundation, which, in collaboration with the pharmaceutical company Ionis, develops individualized antisense oligonucleotide therapies for nano-rare diseases, those whose mutations affect fewer than thirty individuals worldwide. Eligibility requires a confirmed genetic diagnosis and the involvement of a research physician to guide the process. While this path is highly personalized, it involves collaboration between families, researchers, and institutions to ensure feasibility. Importantly, n-Lorem provides these therapies at no cost to patients or families. This initiative highlights how advances in precision medicine are creating possibilities for patients who previously had no treatment options.

Is It a Clinical Trial or a Scam?

Where there's hope, there's often someone trying to take advantage. Sadly, clinical trial scams prey on vulnerable patients. This section will help you spot and avoid them.

Red Flag #1: Unsolicited Emails, Texts, or Links

If you receive an unsolicited email or text inviting you to see if you qualify for a clinical trial, proceed with caution. These links may install malware on your computer or phone, giving scammers access to your personal information, or direct you to fake websites that appear legitimate and ask for sensitive data. Legitimate institutions, such as patient advocacy groups or hospitals, might contact you about a trial, but only if you've previously authorized them to do so. If you're unsure about an email or link, don't click the link, and contact the institution using their official phone number or website to verify the communication. Social media ads about clinical trials can also be misleading. Always double-check the source before engaging.

Red Flag #2: They Ask for Money

Legitimate clinical trials are always free. Many trials provide compensation for your time or travel expenses. If someone asks you to pay for an experimental therapy or to participate in a trial, it's a scam.

🔍 One of the most common scams involves stem cell therapies, often marketed with exaggerated promises. "Stem cell clinics" claim to offer treatments for a wide range of conditions (from Alzheimer's disease to knee pain to post-COVID syndrome) using slick ads and glowing testimonials. Patients may be charged tens of thousands of dollars for unapproved, unproven, and often harmful procedures. These "therapies" might involve injecting cells derived from fat, falsely claimed to be stem cells. Clinics offering these treatments operate worldwide, including in China, Mexico, the Dominican Republic, and even the United States. Some patients have suffered severe complications, including blindness or tumors, while others find that the treatment simply doesn't work, leaving them poorer and no closer to a cure. The FDA has repeatedly warned against these scams.[5]

⚠ Remember, you should never pay for an unapproved experimental therapy.

Red Flag #3: The Trial Is Not Registered

All legitimate clinical trials must be listed in a public registry, such as ClinicalTrials.gov. If a trial isn't listed, it's unlikely to be legitimate.

There are two exceptions to this rule: (i) small trials in countries outside the United States might not appear in ClinicalTrials.gov but could still be listed in local registries (see Table 3.1. above for a list of local registries); (ii) if a Phase 1 trial is exclusively enrolling healthy volunteers, it may not appear in ClinicalTrials.gov either.

⚠ Some illegitimate trials and scams may still appear in registries. You must use your judgment and verify all details. And, as mentioned earlier, ClinicalTrials.gov and the other registries also list research studies that are not clinical trials.

Red Flag #4: Lack of Informed Consent

Legitimate clinical trials require participants to provide informed consent. This process ensures that you understand the study's purpose and procedures, potential risks and benefits, and your rights and responsibilities as a participant. You'll be given a detailed informed consent form to review and sign. If the clinical trial study team skips this step or doesn't provide adequate information, it's a scam (more details on the informed consent in Chapter 5).

To protect yourself from these scams, make sure you:

- Verify All Communications: Only respond to institutions or organizations you trust and have a prior relationship with.
- Use Trusted Registries: Familiarize yourself with ClinicalTrials.gov or other country-specific registries.
- Ask Questions: Don't hesitate to seek clarification about the trial's procedures, compensation, and legitimacy.
- Trust Your Instincts: If something feels off, it's better to walk away than risk your safety or finances.

By staying informed and vigilant, you can navigate the world of clinical trials safely and confidently.

I hope the resources in this chapter have left you feeling more empowered to find clinical trials tailored to your specific condition, stage, and location. For those with rare diseases, the number of active trials at any given time may be limited. While this scarcity can be disheartening, it also has the advantage of simplifying your decision-making process. Conversely, certain conditions, particularly some cancers, may have a vast array of ongoing trials. Navigating through so many options can feel overwhelming. How do you prioritize the most promising trials? That's exactly what we'll dive into in Chapter 4.

Chapter 3 Highlights

- Knowing the specifics of your diagnosis, such as disease stage, histological type, and genetic markers, will refine your search and help identify clinical trials that fit your needs.

- ClinicalTrials.gov remains the most comprehensive resource to find trials but navigating it can be challenging.

- Create a spreadsheet to track trial details including phase, NCT number, and eligibility criteria.

- Patient advocacy groups, hospital websites, and pharmaceutical company platforms sometimes offer tailored trial listings, some with personalized support or advanced search options.

- Some AI tools show promise to find trials, but they are not yet publicly accessible or user friendly for most patients. ChatGPT can offer preliminary guidance but is not a substitute for database searches as it does not have the ability to comprehensively search in ClinicalTrials.gov.

- Be cautious with trial-matching platforms. Free, reputable resources like ClinicalTrials.gov and nonprofit patient advocacy organizations are safer options.

Notes

1. If you are interested in the topic of how AI is reshaping medicine, I recommend Peter Lee, Carey Goldberg, and Isaac Kohane, *The AI Revolution in Medicine: GPT-4 and Beyond* (Pearson, 2023).

2. Harry Klein, Tali Mazor, Ethan Siegel, et al., "MatchMiner: An Open-Source Platform for Cancer Precision Medicine," *NPJ Precision Oncology* 6, no. 69 (2022).

3. Qiao Jin, Zifeng Wang, Charalampos S. Floudas, et al., "Matching Patients to Clinical Trials with Large Language Models," *Nature Communications* 15, no. 1 (2024): 9074.

4. Joseph M. Unger, Riha Vaidya, Dawn L. Hershman, et al., "Systematic Review and Meta-Analysis of the Magnitude of Structural, Clinical, and Physician and Patient Barriers to Cancer Clinical Trial Participation," *Journal of the National Cancer Institute* 111, no. 3 (March 2019): 245–55.

5. *FDA Warning: Important Patient and Consumer Information About Regenerative Medicine Therapies*, https://www.fda.gov/vaccines-blood-biologics/consumers-biologics/consumer-alert-regenerative-medicine-products-including-stem-cells-and-exosomes (March 25, 2025).

4

Choosing the Right Clinical Trial

Now that you know how to find clinical trials, the next step is deciding which trial is the best fit for you. This chapter serves as a practical guide to help you evaluate your options and select the trial that aligns with your medical needs, personal goals, and logistical realities. Choosing a clinical trial can feel overwhelming, especially if you have several to choose from.

This chapter will provide you with tools to navigate this decision-making process effectively. We'll start by outlining the key questions to ask yourself before committing to a trial. Then, we'll explore how to rank trials based on factors such as treatment goals, phase, mechanism of action of the drug, logistics, and potential risks. We'll also delve into considerations like trial location, investigator reputation, and your overall comfort level with the study protocol.

By the end of this chapter, you should feel confident in making an informed choice. Whether you ultimately decide to participate or not, the insights you gain will be invaluable as you take the next steps in your treatment journey.

Key Questions before Selecting a Trial

Before diving into the details of any specific trial, it's crucial to take a step back and ask yourself some foundational questions. These will help clarify your priorities and filter out trials that may not be a good fit.

1. Does the trial align with your health goals? Consider whether the trial's objectives match your priorities. Are you hoping to slow disease progression, manage symptoms, or access cutting-edge experimental treatments? For example, if you have advanced cancer, a trial focused on extending survival might be more appealing than one studying disease mechanisms. Understanding the trial's purpose helps ensure that it aligns with your expectations and goals.

2. What is the trial's primary objective? Every clinical trial has a primary goal, such as determining safety, establishing dosing, or assessing long-term benefits. When considering trials, think about whether the primary objective suits your needs. For instance, Phase 1 trials typically have a primary goal of determining safety and dosing, and they are not usually designed to evaluate whether the drug has clear health-related benefits. If your priority is accessing a treatment that might improve your symptoms or slow the progression of the disease, later-phase trials, such as Phase 2 or Phase 3, may be more appropriate than Phase 1. On the other hand, if you're willing to contribute to scientific research without a guaranteed personal benefit, earlier-phase trials might still be worth exploring.

3. Does the trial have realistic eligibility criteria for you? For instance, if a trial requires a lumbar puncture or a liver biopsy

to determine eligibility, ask yourself if you are willing to undergo such testing. Additionally, consider whether you are willing to make significant changes (e.g., stopping current therapies, as some trials require participants to be off some medications), as these might be required.

4. What is the trial's location and duration? Finding a trial near your home can reduce logistical challenges, but if a promising trial is further away, assess whether you're able to travel for it. Additionally, evaluate the time commitment required. For example, does the trial involve frequent visits or lengthy study visits? Some participants in long-term studies may need to attend follow-ups for years. Ensuring the clinical trial schedule works with your lifestyle can be an important consideration.

5. What are the potential risks and benefits? Every trial has risks. Review the potential risks outlined in the study's informed consent form (more on this in Chapter 5) or ask questions of the study team. On the flip side, assess the trial's potential benefits. Does the trial offer a chance at meaningful improvement in your condition? Or are the benefits more abstract, such as contributing to advancing the science for others?

6. Is the trial well funded and well organized? Trials sponsored by established pharmaceutical companies or reputable not-for-profit organizations often have better resources and infrastructure, which could ensure smoother trial functioning and more support for participants.

⚠ Trials sponsored by smaller biotech companies might still be promising, but it's crucial to do your due diligence to ensure that the company is legitimate, has sufficient funding, and is not involved in questionable practices.

🔍 The biotechnology company Cassava Sciences was once a beacon of hope for Alzheimer's patients. The Phase 2 trial results of its experimental drug, simufilam, were hailed as groundbreaking as it seemed to do the impossible: not just halt, but reverse memory decline. The company quickly launched two Phase 3 trials, enrolling more than 2,000 Alzheimer's patients desperate for treatment. However, behind the scenes, cracks began to show. Whistleblowers and researchers accused Cassava of fabricating data to inflate the drug's efficacy. Investigations by the Department of Justice and the US Securities and Exchange Commission (SEC) revealed widespread scientific misconduct, leading to multi-million-dollar settlement charges and fines for the company and its executives. The ultimate heartbreak came in November 2024, when the Phase 3 results confirmed the doubts: simufilam was not better than placebo. For the Alzheimer's patients and families who had entrusted years of their lives to these trials, it was a betrayal. Instead of progress, they were left with wasted time and shattered hope.

This example underscores the importance of verifying a trial's sponsor, its funding, and the credibility of its scientific claims. Trials with vague or underfunded operations might face logistical challenges, lack participant support, or even risk harming their participants.

Ranking Clinical Trials: How to Prioritize Your Options

Once you've identified several clinical trials that match your condition, stage, and location, the next step is deciding which trial is the best for you. Not all trials are created equal and prioritizing them can be a complex process. Using a structured approach, like the one I propose here, will help you make an informed decision.

Start with a Spreadsheet and Rank the Criteria

As introduced in Chapter 3, a spreadsheet is an excellent tool for organizing information about clinical trials. Use columns for critical data such as the trial's name, NCT number, drug name, inclusion/exclusion criteria, condition or indication, phase, preliminary data, sponsor, and location. This will help you visualize and easily compare your options.

To systematically evaluate and prioritize clinical trials, I recommend a scoring system. In this system, I assign a score from 0 to 3 for each relevant criterion, where 0 indicates the least promising or trustworthy option and 3 represents the best option. While this ranking is arbitrary, I have found that using a wider ranking (i.e., 0 to 4) adds unnecessary complexity while a narrower range (i.e., 0 to 2) provides little differentiation. The 0 to 3 ranking is, in my experience, a balanced option, allowing also to use half points (e.g., giving a score of 1.5 points).

Let's break down the key criteria with practical examples and scores. In the spreadsheet columns I suggested above, the initial data points do not have a ranking. These include the trial's name, NCT number, drug name, and inclusion/exclusion criteria. These fields are mostly for your records and to have the trial localized. The following are the fields that are scored.

Condition or Indication

Trials designed for your specific condition, and even more so for its histological or genetic subtype, are more likely to offer relevant and effective treatments. This specificity has become increasingly important with the rise of targeted therapies, such as antibodies and gene therapies, which often address precise molecular pathways.

For example, imagine you are a sixty-two-year-old woman with locally advanced pancreatic adenocarcinoma, and the cancer has recurred after standard therapy. You live in Los Angeles, California. When entering this information on ClinicalTrials.gov (with the appropriate filters, as discussed in Chapter 3), your search yields sixty-four interventional studies. To make this example more practical, let's focus on two of the sixty-four trials.

Trial NCT05417594 assesses the safety, tolerability, pharmacokinetics, pharmacodynamics, and preliminary efficacy of the experimental drug AZD9574 individually and in combination with anticancer agents in 490 participants with advanced cancer that has recurred/progressed. Note that the condition to be treated here is "advanced cancer that has recurred/progressed." It is enrolling patients with pancreatic cancer, but also any other advanced cancer. So, the specificity for your condition is low. My score is 1. It is not a zero because it is still directed at advanced cancer that has recurred/progressed. It is not a 3, because that would be for a drug highly specific for advanced, recurrent pancreatic cancer. I would use 2 for something of intermediate specificity, like "gastrointestinal cancer" or "any tumor with a specific mutation."

The other trial, NCT05766748, is an open-label study to determine the safety and preliminary evidence of a therapeutic effect of the experimental drug "azeliragon" in patients who are refractory to prior treatment of metastatic pancreatic cancer. This is exactly the type of cancer in our example; however, it is not clear if azeliragon was specifically designed to treat pancreatic cancer (as we will learn later, the answer is no). My score: 2.

The Phase of the Trial

Understanding the trial phase is critical. As explained in Chapter 1, each phase has different goals and characteristics. In Chapter 3 we discussed why a Phase 3 trial might be more appropriate to someone looking for a drug with more evidence of safety and efficacy. However, if no Phase 3 trials are available, don't dismiss an early-phase trial with strong preclinical data or a well-defined mechanism of action specific to your condition.

Both trials in our example (NCT05417594 and NCT05766748) are Phase 1/2 trials, meaning they are in early stage with combined safety and preliminary efficacy objectives. My score for both is 1.5 (reflecting their intermediate stage).

Preliminary Data

Does the experimental drug studied in the trial have any previously published human data (e.g., from early trials in the same indication or other trials in different indications)? If it does, do the results support any promising safety and early efficacy? If human clinical trial data is not available because the drug is in Phase 1, preclinical (animal or cell) study results can also be useful, although the uncertainty is higher as animal efficacy does not always translate into human efficacy.

In our example, trial NCT05417594 uses AZD9574. This code name usually denotes an experimental drug developed by a pharmaceutical company, in this case, the large Swedish-British company AstraZeneca. For people with no scientific and medical background, it can be challenging to decipher whether there is published clinical trial data on such experimental drugs.

💡 Pro Tip: While AI large language model tools are, as of right now, not great at finding active clinical trials (as we discussed in Chapter 3), they are quite effective at digesting complex scientific literature, press releases, and regulatory filings into plain language summaries. This means you can use ChatGPT or other AI chatbots to summarize scientific literature for you. For example, I used the following prompt:

User: "Assume the role of a clinical trial expert who is familiar with ongoing trials and is knowledgeable about scientific databases such as Google Scholar. Can you summarize recent and ongoing research with the experimental drug AZD9574 and whether it has completed Phase 1 or Phase 2 human clinical trials? Your response should be understandable to readers with no scientific or medical background. Your statements should provide enough context to be clear to readers. You should avoid acronyms or measurements unless necessary. It should explain the relevance of the research findings at a level that is understandable to a reader with no scientific or medical background. Your summary should include no more than 200 words."

ChatGPT: *"AZD9574 is an experimental drug being studied for its potential to treat certain types of cancer, particularly brain tumors called gliomas. Gliomas are a type of cancer that starts in the brain or spine and can be very difficult to treat. AZD9574 works by inhibiting an enzyme called PARP1, which is involved in repairing damaged DNA in cancer cells. By blocking this enzyme, AZD9574 can make it harder for cancer cells to repair themselves, potentially leading to their death. Recent research has focused on testing the safety and effectiveness of AZD9574 in combination with another drug called temozolomide. Temozolomide is a chemotherapy drug that is commonly used to treat gliomas. The combination of*

AZD9574 and temozolomide is being studied to see if it can improve treatment outcomes for patients with gliomas that have not responded to other treatments. The clinical trials for AZD9574 are currently in Phase 1 and Phase 2, which means researchers are still evaluating the best dose and assessing the drug's safety and preliminary effectiveness. These trials are ongoing, and researchers are hopeful that AZD9574 could become a valuable new treatment option for patients with difficult-to-treat cancers."

ChatGPT produced an accurate response in clear, accessible language within seconds. AI tools are increasingly valuable for distilling complex scientific information into summaries that are easy for the public to comprehend.[1]

In the other example, trial NCT05766748 uses azeliragon (the fact that the drug has a name and not a code means that it is likely to be in a more advanced stage of development). When I prompted ChatGPT about human data with azeliragon, this is what I got:

ChatGPT: *"Yes, there is human clinical trial data available for azeliragon. Originally developed for Alzheimer's disease, azeliragon was tested in over 2,000 patients in randomized, placebo-controlled trials. While these studies showed the drug was well-tolerated, they did not demonstrate efficacy for Alzheimer's. However, based on its mechanism of action (blocking the receptor for advanced glycation end products, or RAGE), it is now being investigated for glioblastoma and other cancers. Currently, azeliragon is being evaluated in multiple Phase 2 clinical trials for glioblastoma, including one in the*

US for patients with unmethylated glioblastoma and another in Spain combining it with radiation and chemotherapy. Depending on the results, the drug may advance to Phase 3 trials for glioblastoma. Additionally, a Phase 3 trial is ongoing to assess its potential in preventing acute kidney injury in hospitalized pneumonia patients, including those with COVID-19."

So, the drug was initially tested in Alzheimer's patients but is now being investigated in clinical trials for multiple cancers and kidney disease. We discussed drug repurposing in Chapter 1; however, this situation in which multiple indications are being considered without success in any of them resembles a "drug in a desperate search for a disease." This suggests that the biotechnology company is casting a wide net to find any viable application for a molecule already in their pipeline. In my view, this is not an encouraging sign.

My score for both trials is 2, as some animal studies on pancreatic cancer (our condition of interest) have been published (I confirmed this through a scientific literature search, but you could use an AI chatbot).

Sponsor

Trials backed by well-resourced sponsors, such as large pharmaceutical companies, typically benefit from better infrastructure, experienced teams, and robust participant support systems. Smaller biotech companies can also conduct excellent trials, but it's essential to assess their track record and financial stability, as discussed earlier.

In our example, trial NCT05417594 is sponsored by AstraZeneca, one of the largest and most reputable pharmaceutical companies globally. With a proven track record and ample resources, AstraZeneca can successfully manage and complete this trial. My score is a 3 (top score).

Trial NCT05766748, in contrast, is sponsored by Cantex Pharmaceuticals, a small biotech company that lacks a prominent industry presence. A web search reveals that the company is based in Florida and has a limited drug pipeline focused on azeliragon, a compound being tested for multiple unrelated conditions (from cancer to pneumonia and kidney disease, as ChatGPT told us above). This suggests the company is searching for any viable indication for its drug, raising concerns about its focus and strategic direction. If you want to delve deeper into a sponsor's financial stability, public companies often have an "Investors" section on their website, providing access to SEC filings and other financial documents. For private companies, resources like Crunchbase can offer insights into their funding history, investor base, and financial health. In the case of Cantex Pharmaceuticals, a search reveals no major funding rounds, with the company surviving on debt financing. This is a potential red flag for a trial's and the company's long-term viability. My score is a 1.

Location

Decide how far you're willing to travel. Some patients choose trials closer to home for convenience, while others are willing to move for a trial that offers the best chance of success. In Chapter 3 we even discuss the possibility of traveling abroad for trials. You should weigh the potential benefits against the logistical and emotional challenges of participating in a distant trial.

In our examples, both trials are recruiting in Los Angeles, meaning minimal travel. My score: 3 (top score) for both trials.

💡 Pro Tip: Avoid traveling for a Phase 1 clinical trial. These early-stage trials primarily assess safety and dosing, are usually not designed to assess efficacy, and there is a significant chance the drug may not progress to Phase 2 (as discussed in Chapter 1).

Goals and Duration

Examine whether the trial's objectives align with your needs. For example, does the trial aim to slow disease progression, alleviate symptoms, or evaluate long-term survival? Ensure that the trial's focus matches your priorities.

In our example, trial NCT05417594's primary objective is to assess the safety and tolerability of the study drug, which is a standard focus for Phase 1 and Phase 2 trials. Secondary objectives include pharmacokinetic measures, which evaluate how the body processes the drug. This is also typical for these trial phases. Interestingly, some secondary endpoints delve into "progression-free survival," "time to response," and "duration of response," which are more directly linked to slowing disease progression and extending survival. Notably, the study's measurement duration is "approximately three years," long enough to observe meaningful survival effects. Additionally, this is an open-label trial, meaning all participants will receive the study drug. These factors align well with the goals of a pancreatic cancer patient seeking to improve survival through experimental treatment. My score is a 3 (top score).

Trial NCT05766748 lists its primary objective as the "identification of the recommended dose for Phase 2," which is standard for Phase 1 studies. Secondary endpoints include safety, tolerability, "disease control," "overall survival," and "change in performance status." While these endpoints are relevant to survival, the study's short time frame of only eight weeks may not be adequate to observe meaningful effects on these survival-related parameters. Although the trial is open label, meaning all participants will receive the experimental drug, the limited duration significantly reduces its potential to provide actionable insights for a patient seeking long-term benefits. My score is a 1.

Getting the Final Score

Once you've scored each criterion, add up the totals to compare trials:

- Trial NCT05417594 (AZD9574): 12.5 points
- Trial NCT05766748 (azeliragon): 10.5 points

The first trial scores higher due to its well-established sponsor, broader secondary endpoints, and longer duration.

Some criteria may carry more weight for you. For example, you might avoid trials sponsored by lesser-known companies, regardless of other factors. It's okay to prioritize based on your comfort level and instincts.

While the examples here focus on just two trials, you can apply this ranking system to as many trials as necessary. Though it may require a significant investment of time, this method simplifies the decision-making process and ensures that you're prioritizing trials most aligned with your needs.

⚠ Even the highest-ranked trial on your list will test an experimental drug that may or may not be safe or efficacious. Maintaining realistic expectations is essential as you move forward.

💡 Pro Tip: In the rare event that two trials receive the same top score, and you qualify for both, take a strategic approach. If both trials are for the same disease, at the same stage, and conducted at the same research site, consider additional factors like duration. For example, if one trial lasts three months and the other two years, enrolling in the shorter trial may allow you to participate in the longer one later. However, be sure to understand the eligibility criteria carefully. Some trials exclude patients who have received experimental therapies within a certain timeframe (e.g., the past year). Discuss these nuances with the study team to avoid unintended disqualification from future opportunities.

Learning More about the Experimental Therapy and Its Target

When considering a clinical trial, it's crucial to understand not just the experimental treatment but also its target. In medicine, a therapeutic target is the molecule, gene, or pathway the treatment aims to influence to achieve its effects. By grasping what a therapy is targeting, you can better evaluate its potential effectiveness, risks, and mechanisms of action.

What Is a Therapeutic Target?

⚠ A **therapeutic target** is the specific structure in the body that an experimental treatment is designed to interact with to achieve its intended outcome. Targets vary widely, from receptors on cell surfaces to genetic mutations within our DNA, as described in Table 4.1.

Interestingly, many effective drugs lack a fully understood target. Older treatments like lithium (for bipolar disorder) and ketamine (for

Table 4.1 Types of Therapeutic Targets

Target	Definition	Example Target	Example Drug
Receptors	Molecules on cell surfaces that receive signals.	Beta-adrenergic receptors	Propranolol blocks beta-adrenergic receptors to dilate blood vessels thus lowering blood pressure.
Proteins or enzymes	Cellular "workhorses" performing essential tasks.	HMG-CoA reductase	Atorvastatin inhibits HMG-CoA reductase to lower the production of cholesterol.

Target	Definition	Example Target	Example Drug
Genes (DNA)	Our genetic code containing the information for our biological building blocks. Gene therapies can address defective or missing genes to correct genetic disorders.	*SMN1* gene	Zolgensma® replaces the missing *SMN1* gene in SMA.
mRNA	Messenger RNA transmits the information in the DNA to produce proteins. mRNA therapies can instruct cells to block harmful proteins.	*SOD1* mRNA	Tofersen blocks the production of SOD1 protein in patients affected by genetic forms of ALS.
Cellular structures	Physical components within cells, which can also be targets.	Microtubules in cancer cells	Chemotherapy paclitaxel binds to microtubules in cancer cells, hampering their division.

anesthesia and depression) work well despite incomplete knowledge of their mechanisms. Most modern drugs are precisely designed with specific targets in mind, reflecting advances in molecular biology and precision medicine.

Types of Experimental Therapies

Understanding the type of therapy being tested is just as important as knowing its target. Experimental pharmacological therapies generally fall into the therapeutic modalities described in Table 4.2.

Table 4.2 Frequent Therapeutic Modalities

Therapeutic Modality	Definition	Route of Administration	Example
Small molecule	Chemically synthesized drugs that interact with intracellular targets.	Oral	Erlotinib (Tarceva®) inhibits the EGFR protein in certain lung cancers.
Biologics (large molecules): peptides, proteins, or antibodies	Peptides, proteins, or antibodies derived from living organisms.	Parenteral	Insulins like Humalog® regulate blood sugar, while the antibody trastuzumab (Herceptin®) targets HER2 in breast cancer.
Antibody-drug conjugates	Precision therapies combining antibodies targeting specific cells with other drugs (biologics or oligonucleotides).	Parenteral	Brentuximab-vedotin (Adcetris®) delivers chemotherapy directly to cancer cells.
Radioligand therapies	These combine a radioactive isotope with a molecule (ligand) that binds to specific targets, delivering radiation directly to diseased cells.	Parenteral	Lutetium-177 PSMA (Pluvicto®) targets a protein on prostate cancer cells, minimizing damage to surrounding healthy tissue.
Oligonucleotides	RNA molecules that regulate protein production	Parenteral	Nusinersen (Spinraza®) boosts SMN protein for SMA, while patisiran (Onpattro®) silences RNA in hereditary amyloidosis.
Gene therapies	Modify genetic material to treat disease.	Parenteral	Luxturna® treats inherited retinal disease caused by RPE65 mutations.
Cell therapies	Use or modify cells to treat diseases.	Parenteral	CAR-T cell therapy reprograms T-cells to better attack cancer.

Parenteral: any route of administration that is not oral, for instance, intravenous or subcutaneous.

Emerging therapies sometimes defy classification. For instance, microbiome treatments (e.g., fecal transplant for *Clostridium difficile* infection) harness live bacteria to influence health, and drug-coated devices like coronary stents blur the lines between pharmacological and device therapies. Similarly, some device-based interventions, such as deep brain stimulation for Parkinson's disease, target specific brain regions without using drugs.

Understanding the target and type of therapy can help you better evaluate the potential risks and benefits of participating in a clinical trial. By doing your research, asking the right questions, and consulting with your doctor, you'll be better equipped to decide whether a trial aligns with your needs and goals.

💡 Pro Tip: Learning as much as possible about your condition can greatly enhance your ability to evaluate clinical trials. You don't need to become an expert, but a good understanding of your disease and its treatment landscape can help you better grasp the relevance of each clinical trial and the target and mechanisms of action of the experimental drug. For rare and ultra-rare disorders, self-education is even more important, as only a small number of physicians and researchers may be deeply familiar with these conditions. You can use an AI chatbot (e.g., ChatGPT) for this purpose. The following is a potential prompt you could use to learn more about a disease (in this case, e.g., idiopathic pulmonary fibrosis).

User: "Assume the role of a physician-scientist with expertise in pulmonary disorders. Write a summary on idiopathic pulmonary fibrosis, including symptoms, evolution, current treatment options, and any other useful information about the disease. Restrict your sources to scientific articles published in peer-reviewed medical journals. The readers of your summary are patients with this condition who want to learn more about it.

Your readers do not have a medical background, so use plain language and avoid acronyms. Ensure your summary has updated information. Make sure your summary is no longer than 200 words."

You can adjust the prompt based on your preferences. After the initial answer, you can keep asking more specific questions if there are aspects you would like to learn more about.

⚠ If instead of using an AI chatbot, you want to search online directly, stick to reputable sources like known medical organizations or legitimate advocacy groups. While Wikipedia can be interesting for topics such as pop culture or video games, it's unreliable for medical or scientific information. Instead, focus on peer-reviewed literature or trusted organizations for the most accurate and up-to-date knowledge.

🔍 In 1984, Augusto and Michaela Odone received devastating news: their six-year-old son, Lorenzo, was diagnosed with adrenoleukodystrophy (ALD), a rare, fatal neurodegenerative disorder. Doctors gave Lorenzo only a few years to live and no hope of treatment. However, the Odones refused to accept this prognosis. With no medical or scientific background, they immersed themselves in biomedical research. Hours of relentless study led them to develop an oily therapy composed of oleic and erucic acids intended to supplement some of the metabolic deficits caused by ALD. While not a cure, the oil showed promise in slowing disease progression. Their journey was immortalized in the 1992 film *Lorenzo's Oil*, starring Nick Nolte and Susan Sarandon. Thanks to the oil, Lorenzo lived far beyond his initial prognosis, reaching thirty years of age. The Odones' story illustrates how patients' families, armed with determination and access to scientific knowledge, can drive progress in understanding and treating their diseases.

Becoming a Participant in a Clinical Trial

Once you've identified the top-ranked clinical trial that most interests you, the next step is turning your interest into action. Enrolling in a trial is not as straightforward as clicking "sign up"; the process can be complex, bureaucratic, and sometimes frustrating. Here's a step-by-step guide to help you navigate this journey efficiently.

Initiating Contact

Once you've shortlisted trials, the first step is to reach out to the listed contacts on ClinicalTrials.gov (or other registries or websites). These contacts often include clinical trial coordinators, site administrators, or the PI. The contact information often includes their email or phone number.

⚠ Reach out early! If you think you meet the trial's eligibility criteria, reaching out as soon as possible could increase your chances of securing a spot. Once a trial reaches full enrollment, it stops accepting new participants.

To reach out, I would recommend you create and use a standard email template. Draft a clear, polite email explaining your interest in the trial that includes essential details such as your age, diagnosis, and stage of disease. Here is an example template:

Subject: Inquiry about Clinical Trial [enter Trial Name or NCT number] for [enter Disease]

Dear Clinical Trial Team,

I found your clinical trial [enter NCT number] on ClinicalTrials.gov and would like to have more information. I think I might meet the eligibility criteria. My diagnosis is [specific condition], and I am [age]. I am currently located in [city, state]. Would you please let me know if you are still enrolling participants and what additional steps are necessary to participate?

Best wishes,

[Your Name]

[Your email]

[Your phone number]

If they respond right away, great! Some sites may even send you a brochure, leaflet, additional informational materials, or a copy of the informed consent form (ICF) for you to review. The ICF outlines key details about the trial, and while it may include some technical jargon, it's generally written to be understandable to patients. This document is an excellent resource to help you learn more about the trial. We'll explore the ICF in greater detail in Chapter 5.

If you don't receive a response within a week, send a follow-up email. If you still haven't received a reply, try using a different method, such as calling the study site directly or contacting the institution. Persistence can pay off.

Sometimes, the contact information listed might not be accurate. Phone numbers may lead to general hospital lines, and emails may go unanswered. It's not uncommon to encounter errors or dead ends, but don't give up. If the listed phone number or email doesn't work, check the sponsor's official website or call the institution's general line to request the correct contact details for the research team.

If you contacted the clinical trial coordinator and they are unresponsive, consider contacting the PI directly. PIs oversee the study and are often more knowledgeable (and sometimes more responsive!) about trial details. Their contact information is typically found on ClinicalTrials.gov, their institution's website, or published research articles. A quick web search using their name and institution can often yield their contact information.

💡 Pro Tip: Doctor-to-doctor communication can sometimes expedite things. If you're struggling to get a response, consider asking your primary physician to call the trial site on your behalf. Physicians often have an easier time confirming trial status and learning the best way to refer a patient.

If you still don't get a response, consider the following. Many trials are conducted at multiple locations. If one site is unresponsive, try reaching out to another in the same study, even if it's in a different city or state. Sometimes, staff at an alternate site can help connect you with your preferred location or confirm trial availability. If responses remain elusive, consider moving on to the next trial on your spreadsheet.

To make things even more frustrating, you may encounter other inefficiencies, such as outdated listings (trials that appear as "recruiting" on ClinicalTrials.gov may already be full or closed), ineffective waitlists that might not notify you if a spot opens, and variable responses, with some trials requiring you to establish medical care with the hospital or clinic before discussing clinical trial details (more on this in the next section).

Don't despair. Stay proactive, organized, and strategic, and you'll improve your chances of joining a trial that aligns with your needs and goals.

Assessing Preliminary Eligibility: Prescreening

After receiving an initial positive response from the research coordinator, PI, or other clinical trial staff, the next step is assessing your eligibility.

This typically begins with a prescreening, where the trial team reviews your medical records (such as diagnoses, lab results, imaging, and prior treatments) to determine if you meet the basic criteria. Many hospitals and clinics allow you to access and download medical records online through their electronic portals. If online access isn't available, you can ask your doctor's office or hospital records department to send your records directly to the trial site. Under US law (**HIPAA**), you have the right to request your medical records on time. Most requests can be made through a simple form available at your healthcare provider's office or website.

⚠ While US law guarantees your right to access your records, some healthcare providers may charge a reasonable fee for copying and transmitting them. If you face delays or barriers, remind them of your legal rights and inquire about any available fee waivers.

After reviewing your records, the trial team may follow up with additional questions via email or phone to clarify eligibility. Some sites may also request a video call for a more detailed assessment.

For studies requiring a more thorough evaluation, you may need to visit the trial site in person for physical exams, additional lab tests, or imaging.

⚠ Be aware that the prescreening visit may not be part of the clinical trial itself. Some sites may require a separate, standard medical visit to gather necessary information for confirming your diagnosis, which could be billed to your medical insurance. For example, a trial might require participants to have a confirmed diagnosis of a disease, but the trial may not provide the resources or tests needed to establish such diagnosis. In these cases, if your diagnosis is not properly established, the site will need to perform those assessments as part of standard medical care, and these costs may be your responsibility. Make sure to clarify any uncertainties with the trial site to ensure that you understand what costs will be covered and what you may need to arrange or pay for separately.

In other instances, after signing an ICF, the participant may be directly evaluated in the screening visit as part of the clinical trial. We will discuss informed consent and the screening visit in detail in Chapter 5.

Making the Final Decision

Once the study site determines that you meet the preliminary criteria for the trial, you may be scheduled for a screening visit (Chapter 5 provides more information on the screening procedures). This is a critical juncture where you must decide whether to move forward and officially enroll. Once again, evaluate the trial's alignment with your personal goals, medical needs, and lifestyle. Additionally, revisit the broader considerations discussed earlier in this chapter, such as potential risks, benefits, and how the trial fits into your overall care plan.

Finally, don't hesitate to seek input from trusted advisors, your primary physician, loved ones, or even others who have participated in clinical trials. Their perspectives may provide valuable insights to help guide your decision. By taking the time to carefully evaluate all aspects of the trial and its logistics, you can make an informed choice that aligns with your needs and goals.

⚠ Even if you decide to proceed with the trial, you have the right to withdraw at any time, for any reason, or even without providing a reason.

Is Telemedicine Available?

Telemedicine has revolutionized healthcare by allowing patients to consult with specialists across vast distances, but its role in clinical trial enrollment remains underutilized. During the COVID-19 pandemic, federal policies temporarily allowed telemedicine consultations across state lines, significantly improving access. Unfortunately, these allowances have since lapsed, limiting trial participants' ability to engage remotely with study teams located in other states.

For patients unable to travel frequently due to health or logistical constraints, telemedicine could be a lifeline. Allowing initial screening visits or eligibility assessments via video call could save time and resources for both patients and trial teams. While some sites are starting to offer telemedicine for these purposes, others continue to require in-person visits for initial consultations, adding unnecessary strain on patients.

If travel for an in-person visit is challenging, ask the trial team if a telemedicine option is available. Even when telemedicine isn't explicitly mentioned, some sponsors may allow it for patients unable to attend in person. Advocacy for such flexibility could help pave the way for broader adoption of telemedicine in clinical trials.

What Happens If a Trial Is Delayed or Canceled?

Clinical trials are complex, requiring significant planning, coordination, and resources. Delays and cancellations (also known as terminations), though frustrating, are common. For participants with progressive conditions, these disruptions can feel like setbacks but understanding why they occur and how to adapt can help you stay prepared.

The Trial You Selected Is Delayed

Understanding the causes behind these delays and how to navigate them can help you manage expectations and make informed choices.

Imagine you've identified the "perfect" trial on ClinicalTrials.gov. Its status is listed as "Not Yet Recruiting." You contact the site and provide your medical records, and they determine that you're a promising candidate. However, they inform you that the screening visit cannot proceed yet, as enrollment hasn't started. They estimate it will begin in a month and promise to call to schedule your visit. But then eight weeks pass, then ten, then fourteen, and still, no word. Unfortunately, such scenarios are far from rare. Here are the most common reasons for delays:

- Contracting and Site Activation: Before a trial begins at a particular site, a contract must be finalized between the institution and the sponsor, outlining responsibilities and budgets. These negotiations can be lengthy. Once the contract is signed, the sponsor conducts a site activation visit to ensure that all regulatory and operational requirements are in place, involving the PI and key staff.

- Regulatory and Ethical Approvals: Trials require approval from regulatory authorities (e.g., the FDA) and ethics committees, also known as IRBs, before they can begin. Delays often occur if these bodies request changes to the trial design, such as modifying protocols or adding new tests. These adjustments can increase trial costs, necessitate renegotiations with sites, and create a cascading effect of further delays.

- Protocol Amendments: Changes to the trial design, such as adjusting dosing regimens, adding new study endpoints, or modifying eligibility criteria, require amendments to the protocol. These amendments must be approved by regulatory authorities, IRBs, and trial sites, adding time and complexity to the process.

- Manufacturing or Supply Issues: Experimental drugs or devices often require intricate manufacturing processes with stringent quality control standards. Even a minor impurity can trigger quality assurance red flags, halting production until the issue is resolved. These delays can ripple across the trial timeline, particularly if the experimental therapy involves custom components like gene therapies or biologics.

- Funding Shortfalls: Smaller biotech companies or academic sponsors may face financial constraints that interrupt trial operations. Even well-funded organizations can encounter unexpected expenses, such as increased costs due to protocol amendments or delays, which can strain budgets.

- External Factors: Global events like the COVID-19 pandemic, geopolitical conflicts, or natural disasters can disrupt trials on a large scale. For instance, Ukraine was once a leading country for international clinical trial enrollment but has experienced a sharp decline due to the ongoing war. Such unforeseen circumstances can affect recruitment, logistics, and site operations, creating widespread disruptions.

The Trial You Selected Is Terminated

It's also possible that you've successfully qualified for a trial in a prescreening assessment, or even completed the screening visit, or even started receiving the trial drug, only to be notified weeks later that the trial has been canceled. You may be instructed to stop taking the study drug and return to the site for an early termination visit. This can be shocking and disheartening, but it is not unheard of. Trials may end prematurely for several reasons, including:

- Negative Preliminary Data: Early analyses may reveal that the drug or device is either unsafe or unlikely to be effective (futile). In such cases, trials are terminated early to avoid exposing participants to unnecessary risks. Not terminating the trial would be unethical!

- Lack of Funding: Clinical trials are resource intensive. If sponsors are unable to secure the necessary financial support, the trial may be discontinued, even if the experimental therapy shows promise.

- Strategic Shifts: Pharmaceutical companies may choose to reprioritize their pipelines, shelving certain projects midway. This doesn't necessarily indicate the drug is unsafe or ineffective but reflects a strategic decision to focus on other, potentially more lucrative or promising treatments.

- Regulatory Intervention: Regulatory authorities like the FDA may halt a trial if significant safety concerns or compliance issues are identified. This can include alarming safety signals, improper conduct at trial sites, or even suspicions of fabricated data.

What To Do If Your Trial Is Delayed or Terminated

While delays and terminations can feel like dead ends, they are often part of the iterative process of scientific discovery. Even data obtained from terminated trials contributes valuable knowledge that informs future research and improves patient outcomes. Staying flexible, informed, and proactive ensures that you remain in the best position to benefit from ongoing and future advancements.

- Stay Informed: Ask the trial site to keep you updated on the status of the trial, especially if you suspect delays. Inquire about their plans in case the trial timeline shifts.

- Explore Alternatives: If a trial is delayed or canceled, revisit your list of other trials (you should always have your spreadsheet ready!). Keep backups in mind and be prepared to pivot quickly.

- Engage with Advocacy Groups: For rare or specific conditions, advocacy organizations can provide updates on other ongoing research efforts and trials.

- Evaluate Next Steps with Your Doctor: Delays or cancellations are disappointing, but they can also be a chance to reassess treatment options with your healthcare provider.

Chapter 4 Highlights

- Before committing to a trial, evaluate its eligibility criteria, location, and logistics to ensure that it aligns with your medical needs and personal priorities.

- Use a structured ranking system to evaluate trials based on whether the trial is specific to your condition, the phase, the availability of preliminary human data, the sponsor, the location, and the goals and duration.

- Learn about the experimental therapy's mechanism of action and target to better assess its potential benefits and risks.

- Be proactive, persistent, and strategic when contacting trial sites, prepare your medical records, and understand the prescreening and screening processes.

- Delays or cancellations can occur due to regulatory, funding, or safety reasons. Staying informed, having backup options, and consulting with your doctor can help mitigate these challenges.

Note

1   David M. Markowitz, "From Complexity to Clarity: How AI Enhances Perceptions of Scientists and the Public's Understanding of Science," *PNAS Nexus* 3, no. 9 (September 2024): 387.

5

Inside the Clinical Trial: What to Expect

You've identified a clinical trial you might qualify for, contacted the site, submitted your medical records, and got your first visit on the calendar. Congratulations on reaching this important milestone!

Enrolling in a clinical trial is more than just a medical decision; it's a deeply personal step, shaped by hope, determination, and the desire to improve your life. But it's also a personal commitment that requires understanding the process, weighing your options, and preparing for what lies ahead. It's natural to feel a mix of excitement, anticipation, and uncertainty as you prepare to navigate this unfamiliar terrain.

This chapter serves as your guide through the key aspects of trial participation, from your first visit (**screening**), including the informed consent, to your rights and responsibilities and what to expect at each stage. Clinical trials operate under structured protocols designed to test new treatments while prioritizing participant safety. Knowing how the process works will help you approach your trial experience with confidence and clarity.

Clinical research is a partnership between participants and investigators built on trust, transparency, and a shared goal of advancing medicine. By understanding the logistics, expectations, and potential challenges, you'll be better equipped to make informed decisions, advocate for yourself, and navigate this journey with greater ease.

The Informed Consent Is the First Step of the Screening

Your first clinical trial visit, known as the screening visit, is a pivotal step. This is when the trial team confirms that you meet the eligibility criteria to participate in the study. While you may already have an idea of your eligibility based on your medical records or prescreening conversations, the screening visit includes a more rigorous and formal evaluation, which may take several hours, so be patient.

The first step of the screening visit is the informed consent process, which is one of the most important steps when joining a clinical trial.

While signing the ICF is essential, it should be the final step in a thoughtful and thorough process. Informed consent is more than just a signature; it's about ensuring you fully understand what participating in the trial entails and feel confident about your decision to proceed.

The Informed Consent Process

The FDA and other regulatory agencies require that every clinical trial participant provide written consent before enrolling in a study.

📖 **Informed Consent Process**: A continuous, interactive discussion between the study team and the participant, ensuring that the individual fully understands the trial's purpose, risks, and potential benefits before deciding to enroll. The process goes beyond signing a form; it includes ongoing communication throughout the study, allowing participants to ask questions and reaffirm their willingness to continue at any stage.

📖 **Informed Consent Form (ICF)**: A legal document that provides potential clinical trial participants with detailed information about the study, including its purpose, procedures, risks, benefits, and alternative options. By signing the ICF, a participant confirms they have received and understood this information and voluntarily agree to take part in the trial. However, signing the form does not waive a participant's rights, and they may withdraw from the study at any time.

Most clinical trials still rely on traditional paper forms for informed consent. However, electronic and video consent formats are becoming increasingly common, offering more accessible, interactive, and convenient ways for participants to review study details.

⚠ If a study team skips the informed consent process or fails to provide an ICF, walk away immediately. A legitimate trial will always prioritize transparency and the participants' rights. Any deviation from this process is a serious warning sign that the study may be unethical or even fraudulent.

The informed consent process ensures that you have all the necessary information to make an educated choice about participation. It begins with an introduction to the study, usually led by the PI or another key member of the study team, such as the clinical trial coordinator. This is your opportunity to ask questions, express concerns, and clarify any doubts. The study team should clearly explain the purpose of the trial, the experimental nature of the treatment, and your responsibilities as a participant.

Take your time to read the ICF. If needed, take it home and discuss it with your family, caregivers, or primary healthcare provider.

💡 Pro Tip: Bring a written list of questions with you. This ensures that you cover all your concerns during the discussion. Here's a list of potential questions to consider asking during the informed consent process:

- About the trial:
    - What is the primary goal of this study?
    - Why is this trial important to me?
    - How long will the trial last?
    - How many visits will I need to attend, and what is expected at each visit?
    - Could I receive the experimental therapy after the trial ends?
    - Has this study been reviewed and approved by an independent review board?
    - Will I be informed of the study results?

- About the experimental therapy:
    - What is the therapy, and how does it work?
    - Has it been tested in humans before?
    - Is this drug approved in other countries or for other diseases?
    - What are the chances that it will work?
    - What are the known risks or side effects in people (or animals)?
    - Who is sponsoring this trial? Is it a big pharmaceutical company or a small biotech?
    - If I choose not to participate in this trial, what are the alternatives?

- About your responsibilities:
    - Are there lifestyle restrictions (e.g., avoiding certain medications, foods, or activities)?

- What happens if I miss a visit or need to withdraw from the study?
  - How much of my time will the study take?
- About costs and compensation:
  - Will there be any costs to me for participating in this trial?
  - Is there compensation for my time and travel expenses?
- About privacy and confidentiality:
  - How will my data be protected?
  - Will my information or samples be shared with other researchers?
- Other practical questions:
  - Who do I contact if I have questions or experience side effects?
  - If genetic testing is involved, will I have the option to see my results?
  - Could you send the results of my bloodwork or imaging tests to my primary care physician?
  - What is the principal investigator's background and training? How many studies has he or she conducted before?
  - Does the investigator have any financial interest in the drug being studied? What is the relationship between the investigator and the pharmaceutical company sponsoring the trial?

🔍 Grapefruit is often mentioned in ICFs as a prohibited fruit in clinical trials because it can interfere with drug metabolism, leading to inconsistent or harmful effects. This is due to its impact on enzymes that play a key role in metabolizing many drugs. A notable incident occurred during a cholesterol-lowering drug trial, where participants who consumed grapefruit juice experienced unexpected spikes in drug levels, resulting in side effects like muscle pain and liver enzyme elevations. To avoid such interactions and ensure reliable results, researchers typically advise participants to avoid grapefruit products.

⚠ If you're unclear about any aspect of the trial, ask the study team for clarification. There's no such thing as a "bad" question.

How Easy (or Difficult) Is It to Understand the Informed Consent Form?

The ICF should provide a comprehensive overview of the study. While efforts are ongoing to make ICFs shorter and more accessible to the public, summarizing all the necessary information, including technical terms, remains a challenge. This means that going through the ICF may still feel overwhelming as the form may be long and full of scientific jargon.

According to the 2023 *Perceptions and Insights Study* by CISCRP, which surveyed more than 2,000 recent clinical trial participants, the length of the ICF varied widely.[1] Participants reported that their most recent ICF was:

- 1 to 5 pages: 31 percent
- 6 to 10 pages: 22 percent
- 11 to 20 pages: 15 percent
- More than 20 pages: 10 percent

In the same survey, over 90 percent of participants stated that they found the ICF either "very easy" or "somewhat easy" to understand.

Taking the time to read the ICF and asking questions is always worth it.

What's Inside the Informed Consent Form?

Here's what you can expect to find inside the ICF:

- Study Overview: The purpose of the trial and its experimental nature and a summary of the study's goals and key objectives.

- Visit Schedule and Procedures: A breakdown of the duration of the study, the visits, including the tests, imaging, questionnaires, or procedures at each stage, with specific details about invasive procedures, such as the amount of blood drawn (e.g., milliliters or tablespoons) or imaging techniques used.

- Potential Risks and Discomforts: Potential side effects of the drug or therapy based on preclinical or earlier clinical data, and how these side effects will be managed by the trial team.

- Potential Benefits: The expected positive outcomes for you as a participant (if any), or, at least, the broader benefits to future patients or the scientific community.

- Confidentiality and Data Use: How your data will be collected, stored, and used, whether your data or samples can be used in future studies, and whether they will be anonymized.

- Genetic Testing (if applicable): If genetic testing is part of the trial, the ICF should state whether you'll have the option to know your results.

- Costs and Compensation: Clearly outlines that participation should not incur any costs to you and states whether you will receive compensation or reimbursement for travel expenses.

- Contact Information: A phone number or email for questions during the trial or in case of adverse events.

- Signatures: A space for your signature and the investigator's signature to confirm mutual agreement once all your questions have been answered and you are ready to proceed with the screening visit.

The informed consent document can sometimes include dense or technical language. To ensure that you fully understand, consider asking the study team to summarize key points, especially regarding risks and benefits; request simplified examples or scenarios that illustrate what participating will involve; and bring a trusted friend, family member, or caregiver to help you evaluate the information.

Signing the Informed Consent Form

Once all your questions have been answered and you have confirmed your willingness to enroll in the trial, you will be asked to sign the ICF.

⚠ If you're not ready to sign the document yet, that's perfectly fine. Take the document home, review it thoroughly, and discuss it with your loved ones or your doctor. While you won't be able to proceed with the screening visit without signing the ICF, your participation must come from a place of free and fully informed decision-making. It's far better to take your time and fully understand the trial than to commit without clarity or confidence. Remember, this is your choice, you're the one volunteering, and it's essential that you feel empowered and informed every step of the way.

By signing the ICF, you acknowledge that you understand and accept the known risks involved in the trial. This is not a mere formality; it is a critical step in ensuring your autonomy and informed decision-making. Importantly, providing your consent does not absolve the PI, the study team, or the sponsor of their legal and ethical obligations to safeguard your safety and provide professional care throughout the trial. Nor does it waive your right to take legal action in the event of negligence or unlawful conduct. However, by consenting, you accept that you have been fully informed of the known risks, and if a risk explicitly outlined in the ICF occurs, it may be argued that you were aware of its possibility.

After signing the ICF, the study team should provide you with a copy for your records. This document serves as an important reference throughout the trial. If English is not your primary language, ask if a translated version of the ICF is available. Many clinical trials offer ICFs in multiple languages to ensure that all participants fully understand the document.

It's important to recognize that the informed consent process is not a one-time event that ends the moment you sign the ICF. Instead, it's an ongoing process that continues throughout your participation in the trial. The study team is responsible for regularly updating you about the trial's progress, any changes in procedures, or new information that may affect your decision to continue. If they don't proactively provide updates or explanations, you have every right to ask questions and expect clear, thorough answers.

If you feel that the research team has not adequately answered your questions, you have additional options. You could contact the IRB that approved the trial. The IRB's contact information is typically included in the ICF. Alternatively, you could reach out to the pharmaceutical company sponsoring the trial. Many sponsors have consumer helplines specifically for trial-related questions or concerns. Their helpline number should be included in the ICF, or you may find it on the web.

⚠ Signing the ICF does not obligate you to remain in the trial. You are free to withdraw at any time, for any reason, or even for no reason, without penalty or loss of access to standard care. This autonomy is central to your rights as a trial participant.

The informed consent process is your chance to become a fully informed participant. Taking the time to understand the ICF and asking questions ensures that you're not just signing a document but actively agreeing to participate in a way that aligns with your values, goals, and comfort level. This is your choice, and the study team is there to support you every step of the way.

Exceptions to the Rules

When the participant cannot provide consent due to age or cognitive impairment (e.g., young children, individuals with advanced dementia), a parent, caregiver, or legal guardian may sign the ICF on their behalf. In these cases, it is critical that the designated proxy fully understands the study, its potential risks and benefits, and the participant's rights. For example, a parent might provide consent for a pediatric leukemia trial, or a legal guardian might consent on behalf of a person with severe Alzheimer's disease.

In rare and tightly regulated scenarios, the FDA permits research to begin without prior informed consent. This typically applies in emergencies where immediate intervention is necessary and obtaining consent is not feasible. For instance, a patient arriving at the emergency department unconscious due to cardiac arrest may be enrolled in a resuscitation trial testing a new lifesaving intervention. These exceptions are only permissible when

- the medical condition being studied is life threatening,
- existing treatments are ineffective or inadequate, and
- the research offers the potential for direct benefit to the participant.

Additionally, as with any trial, the research protocol must have received prior approval from an IRB and included a community consultation process to inform the public about the study. Once the participant stabilizes, or a family member is available, informed consent is sought retroactively to continue participation. If the participant or family member does not wish to proceed, the individual can be withdrawn from the study.

These exceptions demonstrate the balance that clinical trials must strike between advancing critical research and safeguarding participant rights. They underline the importance of robust oversight to ensure that even in exceptional cases, ethical standards are maintained.

Understanding Trial Criteria and Confirming Eligibility

After the informed consent is thoroughly discussed, your questions answered, and the ICF signed, the other assessments of the screening visit can take place. These typically include the following.

Medical History and Records Review

Be prepared to discuss your full medical history, including diagnoses, treatments (past and current), medications (as well as vitamins and supplements), and surgeries. If you haven't already provided copies of your relevant medical records, bring them with you. This can help streamline the process and avoid delays.

Physical Examination

Most trials require a general physical exam. Depending on the condition being studied or the experimental treatment's expected side-effect profile, the exam may include more detailed assessments. For instance, if the drug could cause peripheral neuropathy (e.g., pins and needles, numbness, or related symptoms), the trial team might conduct a thorough neurological exam.

Tests and Assessments

Blood tests, imaging scans, or other procedures are typically required to assess your overall health status and identify any underlying conditions that could pose risks during the trial. These tests may include renal and liver function assessments, even if you have no known history of issues in these areas. For example, if screening reveals early kidney dysfunction, you might be deemed ineligible for the trial but recommended to follow up with your primary doctor. You might also qualify for a different trial with less stringent renal criteria.

⚠ Remember: while many screening-related tests are covered by the trial sponsor, some medical evaluations may be considered part of establishing care and billed to your insurance. For instance, if the trial requires confirmation of your diagnosis through specialized imaging but does not include such imaging test as part of the screening, the site might bill your insurer for these tests. Always ask about potential costs upfront to avoid surprises.

Diagnostic Confirmation

For some trials, specific diagnostic details must be verified, such as biomarkers, genetic mutations, or disease severity. For example, a trial for metastatic breast cancer may require confirmation of HER2 expression, or a neurology trial might necessitate brain imaging or cerebrospinal fluid collection through a spinal tap.

Questionnaires

The screening visit may include a range of questionnaires designed to assess various aspects of your condition, such as symptoms, well-being, quality of life, and the burden of disease. In some cases, these questionnaires may also involve input from your caregiver to provide a broader perspective on your health and daily challenges.

Completing these questionnaires can sometimes take several hours. While the process may feel tedious, the information collected is key for the trial team to establish a comprehensive **baseline** and better understand your individual needs and circumstances. Patience and thoroughness during this step can significantly contribute to the trial's success.

Inclusion and Exclusion Criteria

Every clinical trial is guided by a strict set of eligibility criteria, rules that determine who can participate. These criteria serve two essential purposes: ensuring the safety of participants and maintaining the scientific integrity of the study. While they may seem like bureaucratic red tape, these rules protect participants and ensure that the trial produces reliable and meaningful results.

Eligibility criteria are divided into two categories:

- **Inclusion Criteria:** These are the conditions you must meet to qualify for the trial. For example, a trial for Alzheimer's might require participants to be aged sixty to eighty with no history of other neurological diseases.

- **Exclusion Criteria:** These are the conditions that disqualify you from participating. Using the same Alzheimer's example, you might be excluded if you have a history of uncontrolled hypertension or are currently receiving medications that interact with the experimental drug.

⚠ Most inclusion and exclusion criteria are nonnegotiable and absolute and there is no wiggle room. However, a few may include qualifiers such as "in the opinion of the investigator." This allows some flexibility, giving the trial's PI discretion to assess whether you meet the spirit of the criteria. For example, a criterion might state: "Participants must be in generally good health, in the opinion of the investigator." This subjectivity can sometimes work in favor of borderline candidates.

Eligibility criteria are intentionally narrow to control variables that might affect the study outcomes. This ensures that any observed effects are likely due to the experimental treatment rather than external factors. For example:

- A trial testing a new asthma medication may exclude participants with smoking-related lung damage because their condition could interfere with the results.
- A trial for a Parkinson's treatment might include only those in the early stages of the disease to assess the drug's potential to slow progression, excluding those with advanced disease.

In some cases, the screening process might extend over several days. For example, on the first day, you might sign the ICF, complete blood tests, questionnaires, and a physical examination, while imaging studies are conducted on a subsequent day. Before attending your visit, ask the trial team about the schedule, time commitment, and expectations.

Once all the procedures are completed, the study team will determine whether you fulfill the eligibility criteria. However, if some tests require centralized analysis or interpretation (common with specialized imaging or biomarkers), it may take several days or even weeks for results to return. The screening period can sometimes extend up to two months, particularly if complex or experimental tests are involved. This gap between the screening and the next visit, often the randomization visit, allows the team to compile and review all results.

⚠ Stay in regular contact with the trial site after your screening visit to ensure that all your results are received and your eligibility is confirmed. Proactively following up can help you secure a date for the next visit without unnecessary delays. Timely communication during this phase is essential to avoid prolonging the process.

Your screening visit is not just about confirming eligibility. It's also an opportunity for you to ask questions, understand what's involved, and ensure that the trial is a good fit for you. This critical step sets the stage for your participation in the study, helping you transition confidently into the next phase of the clinical trial journey.

What Is a Screen Failure?

Even if you thought that you met the eligibility criteria on paper, you may not make it past the initial screening visit. This is referred to as a **screen failure** and occurs when additional tests or assessments reveal that you don't fully meet the trial requirements.

For instance, you might apply for a trial requiring participants to have hemoglobin levels of at least 12 g/dL. If your lab results during screening show 11.9 g/dL, you'd fail the screening process. While frustrating, this process ensures that the trial remains safe and scientifically rigorous.

In some (but not all) cases, a participant who fails the initial screening may be eligible for rescreening, especially if the issue causing the screen failure is temporary and can be resolved. For example, a participant with mild anemia may qualify for rescreening after treatment to raise their hemoglobin levels; or someone with slightly elevated blood pressure might be reconsidered if their hypertension is stabilized with medication.

⚠ Rescreening is at the discretion of the investigator and depends on the study protocol. Not all trials permit rescreening. If you experience a screen failure, don't hesitate to ask whether rescreening is an option for you.

⚠ Being accepted into a clinical trial is not guaranteed. Potential candidates can be excluded for reasons such as age, the stage of their disease, coexisting conditions, or simply because the trial has already reached its recruitment target. But don't be discouraged. Instead, return to your physician, reach out to patient advocacy groups, and revisit the spreadsheet you created to track eligible trials. Keep refining your search as new opportunities may arise.

After the Screening: Randomization and Additional Visits

Once you've completed the screening process and met the eligibility criteria, the next critical step is often the baseline or randomization visit. This marks the start of your participation in the trial as a study subject and sets the stage for evaluating the treatment's impact.

The baseline visit typically includes the randomization (introduced in Chapter 2), especially in controlled trials. This process assigns participants to study groups (such as the treatment group receiving the experimental therapy or the control group receiving a placebo or standard care) through a randomized method designed to eliminate bias. This ensures the study's scientific validity and fairness.

Randomization isn't always a 1:1 split between treatment and placebo groups. Many studies use asymmetrical randomization (e.g.,

2:1 or 3:1) to increase the odds of receiving the experimental treatment. If you have concerns about group assignments, discussing these with the study team can help set realistic expectations. Remember, participants and researchers typically remain blinded to assignments in double-blind studies to preserve objectivity.

The baseline visit establishes your starting point for the trial, and all future measurements will be compared against the data collected during this visit, not the screening visit. For instance, in an Alzheimer's disease trial evaluating cognitive outcomes, your baseline cognitive tests will serve as the reference point to assess any changes. This visit often involves:

- Comprehensive Evaluations: Many of the tests, examinations, or questionnaires completed during screening may be repeated, including the reconfirmation that you fulfill all the inclusion criteria and do not meet any of the exclusion criteria. This ensures uniformity in measurements and eliminates variability between different time points.

- Protocol-Specific Assessments: Some protocols allow the use of recent screening visit data if it aligns with baseline requirements and the visits occur close together. However, if significant time has passed, tests may need to be repeated.

- First Dose of Study Drug: For trials testing oral medications, participants may take the first dose of the study drug (or placebo) under supervision at the study site. If required, you'll likely remain under observation for a few hours to monitor for any immediate side effects.

After the baseline and randomization visit, you'll likely return home and follow a structured schedule for subsequent visits. These follow-ups are essential for monitoring your health, assessing drug effects, and collecting data for the trial. The frequency and nature of these visits depend on the trial protocol and may include:

- Medical Checkups: Regular evaluations to monitor your overall health and detect any adverse effects.
- Lab Tests: Periodic bloodwork or imaging to assess the drug's efficacy and safety.
- Questionnaires: Ongoing symptom, quality of life, and other assessments to gauge treatment impact.
- Dosing or Interventions: Depending on the protocol, additional doses of the study drug may be administered.

With the growing adoption of telemedicine, many trials now include virtual visits, enabling certain assessments to be completed from the comfort of your home. However, some tests, such as imaging or blood draws, may still require in-person visits.

For participants, it is key to:

1. Understand the Schedule: Ensure that you have a clear understanding of the trial schedule, including the number, frequency, and location of visits.
2. Logistics: Plan for transportation and potential overnight stays if the trial site is far from home.
3. Stay in Communication: Maintain regular contact with the study team and notify them of any changes in your availability or health.

⚠ Missing scheduled visits or failing to adhere to the protocol can affect trial outcomes and may lead to your removal from the study. Always communicate with the study team to address any scheduling conflicts or personal challenges.

Participants' Responsibilities and Commitment

Signing the ICF and joining a clinical trial involves not only the opportunity to contribute to groundbreaking medical research but also the acceptance of certain responsibilities. Being aware of these commitments can help participants make an informed decision and enhance the trial's success. If you fail to meet these obligations, the data collected during the clinical trial may be useless.

Following the Study Protocol

The study protocol is a meticulously designed blueprint outlining every aspect of the trial, including what participants need to do: attending scheduled visits, adhering to treatment regimens, and completing assessments such as questionnaires or diaries. This framework ensures the study's integrity and the reliability of its results. Noncompliance with the protocol can endanger your safety and compromise the validity of the trial outcomes.

For example, missing multiple blood-draw appointments may render your data incomplete, potentially leading to your exclusion from the study's final analysis. Or suppose a trial is studying the effects of an experimental medication on blood sugar levels, and participants are required to follow a specific diet. If participants deviate from this diet without reporting it, the resulting data might not accurately reflect the medication's effects. This could lead to incorrect conclusions about the drug's safety or efficacy.

Following the protocol diligently is not only a personal responsibility but also a commitment to the success of the trial and to advancing medical research that may benefit others in the future.

Communicating Truthfully and Honestly

Open and truthful communication with the study team is essential for your safety and the integrity of the clinical trial. Regardless of how much you want to participate, honesty is nonnegotiable. Omitting important details, such as prior medical conditions or current pain treatments, may seem harmless, but it could disqualify you and compromise the trial's accuracy. Worse, some individuals attempt to participate in two trials simultaneously, something strictly prohibited. This can be extremely dangerous, as taking two experimental drugs at the same time may lead to unpredictable interactions, potentially resulting in severe health issues or even death.

Equally important is reporting any changes during the trial, such as new side effects, symptoms, medications, or lifestyle habits. These updates help researchers monitor your safety and the drug's efficacy, ensuring that the trial's goals are met responsibly and accurately.

🔍 Clinical trials investigating the psychedelic psilocybin for anxiety and depression in cancer patients faced challenges related to the participants' motivation to join the studies. For example, some participants had prior experience using psychedelics recreationally, which could influence their expectations and outcomes during the study. Thus, a significant proportion of these participants likely joined the trials specifically to have free access to psilocybin for its hallucinogenic effects rather than for its therapeutic potential or scientific altruism. Moreover, participants and study staff could often deduce whether they had received the active dose based on the drug's hallucinogenic effects, complicating efforts to maintain a true placebo-controlled design. This bias not only influenced the study's outcomes but also led some participants to withdraw early if they suspected they had received a placebo, believing the trial no longer served their interests of getting free "trips." These participants clearly had the wrong motivations to participate in clinical trials, which is one of the reasons that, in June 2024, an expert committee at the FDA advised against using psilocybin for PTSD.

Maintaining Consistency

Participants in clinical trials are often required to follow strict guidelines regarding diet, medications, and lifestyle to ensure reliable study results and safeguard their health. For example, certain foods like grapefruit (as discussed earlier) or beverages such as alcohol may be prohibited because they can interfere with drug metabolism.

Additionally, many trials require that participants maintain a stable medication regimen, meaning they cannot start new medications, adjust doses, or add supplements without approval from the study team. Even minor changes can introduce variability, making it difficult to determine whether a drug is effective or causing side effects.

⚠ Failing to disclose a new medication or supplement, for example, could interfere with the study results by masking side effects or distorting the data. Transparency at every stage is not just a personal obligation, it's a critical part of contributing to the advancement of medical science.

Failure to adhere to these requirements can lead to a **protocol deviation**, which could compromise the integrity of the study and, in some cases, result in withdrawal from the trial. Researchers aim to minimize confounding factors, ensuring that any observed effects are due to the study drug, not external influences.

If you ever find yourself struggling to adhere to a study requirement, it's best to communicate openly with the research team rather than risk noncompliance. They may be able to offer solutions or determine whether an adjustment is possible within the protocol.

Attending Scheduled Visits

Clinical trials involve multiple visits for treatments, monitoring, and follow-ups. Missing appointments can delay data collection and jeopardize the study's progress.

⚠ If you cannot attend an already scheduled trial visit, contact the study team immediately to determine the best course of action. Sometimes, it might be possible to get some of the bloodwork locally or have some of the assessments performed via telemedicine.

Completing Questionnaires and Diaries

Many clinical trials require participants to regularly complete diaries, surveys, or questionnaires to track symptoms, medication adherence, side effects, and overall quality of life. These may be recorded daily, weekly, or at specific intervals throughout the study.

While these tasks can sometimes feel repetitive or tedious, they can be crucial for assessing the real-world impact of the treatment. Unlike lab tests or imaging, self-reported data provides insight into how a drug affects daily functioning, such as sleep, mood, energy levels, or pain levels.

Some trials use paper diaries, while others rely on electronic tablets, apps, or wearable devices that prompt participants to enter data at specific times. Ensuring accuracy and consistency is important as incomplete or delayed entries can compromise the study's findings.

If you miss an entry or struggle with the process, notify the trial staff. They can provide guidance, troubleshoot technical issues, or clarify what's most important to record. Ultimately, your input plays a key role in shaping how new treatments are evaluated and approved.

Keeping Study Drug and Supplies Safe

Participants in clinical trials involving experimental drugs, devices, or home-use kits must follow storage and usage instructions meticulously. For example, if medications need refrigeration, it's crucial to store them accordingly to maintain their potency and effectiveness. Devices and treatments should only be used as directed to ensure accurate results and participant safety.

⚠ Never attempt to alter or tamper with the experimental medication, whether that involves opening syringes, capsules, or devices, as it can compromise both the study's integrity and your health.

🔍 In one placebo-controlled trial I led as PI, two participants who had completed the screening process and been randomized violated the study's blinding protocol. Both participants had received identical capsules, one containing the active drug and the other a placebo. As a double-blind study, neither the participants nor the study team knew which was which. However, these participants had met through a patient advocacy group, become friends, and decided to "investigate." They got together and opened their capsules, discovering that one contained white powder and the other red powder. Correctly deducing that one was taking the active drug and the other the placebo (even though they did not know which one was which), they unknowingly compromised the integrity of the trial. When the study team uncovered this breach, both participants were immediately removed from the trial: a necessary but difficult decision. For the participants, it meant losing the opportunity to continue receiving an experimental therapy that might have helped slow the progression of their disease. Although they did not definitively determine which capsule contained the drug and which the placebo, their actions could have compromised the trial's integrity. For instance, if one participant experienced adverse effects while the other did not, they might infer their respective assignments, introducing bias into the study results.

Notifying the Study Team about Changes

Life doesn't pause for a clinical trial. Major life events, such as relocating, changing jobs, travel plans, or unexpected health issues, can impact your ability to follow study requirements. If any significant changes occur, it's essential to notify the study team as soon as possible.

Some trials have some flexibility built into their protocols. Depending on the situation, the research team may be able to adjust appointment schedules to accommodate work or travel, arrange for lab work or assessments at a different site if you're relocating, modify communication methods, such as shifting to virtual check-ins, and provide guidance on safely continuing or withdrawing if participation becomes too difficult.

Failure to inform the study team could lead to protocol deviations that may compromise both your safety and the integrity of the trial. If withdrawal is necessary, doing so in a structured way ensures that you receive proper medical follow-up and that your contributions to the study remain valid. Keeping the study team informed allows them to support you while ensuring the trial's success.

Understanding Long-Term Commitments

Some studies require long-term follow-ups even after the treatment phase ends. These follow-ups are crucial for understanding the treatment's long-term safety and efficacy. Participants should be prepared for this commitment when enrolling.

By understanding and accepting these responsibilities, participants can ensure that they contribute meaningfully to the research while safeguarding their health and well-being. This mutual commitment between the participant and the study team is essential to advancing medical knowledge and bringing new treatments to light.

What Happens If You Want to Stop Your Participation in a Trial?

Participating in a clinical trial is entirely voluntary, and you retain the right to withdraw (i.e., stop) at any time and for any reason, or even for no reason at all. This is a fundamental right of any study participant. You should never feel coerced to stay in the trial if you've decided to leave. However, withdrawing is a significant decision that requires thoughtful consideration and clear communication with the study team. If leaving the trial could potentially harm you, for instance, by abruptly stopping treatment, the study investigator is obligated to inform you of these risks.

Importantly, withdrawing from a trial should not impact your right to receive medical care from the same physician or institution. Moreover, you are entitled to be informed of any critical developments related to the experimental drug, particularly if they might affect your health.

According to the 2023 *Perceptions and Insights Study* by CISCRP, which surveyed more than 4,500 past clinical trial participants, 10 percent of participants chose to withdraw from a trial before their final visit.[2] The reasons for early withdrawal varied, but the most common included:

- experiencing too many side effects (15 percent);
- personal or logistical challenges, such as difficulty traveling to study sites (14 percent);
- poor communication with the clinical trial team (12 percent);

- finding trial procedures too burdensome, such as frequent testing (12 percent); or
- lack of virtual visit options, making participation more difficult (12 percent)

These findings highlight the diverse challenges participants face and emphasize the importance of clear communication, logistical support, and flexible trial designs to improve retention.

If you decide to withdraw, it's crucial to do so in a way that minimizes disruption to the study and ensures your safety:

1. Notify the Study Team: Inform the research team of your decision and share your concerns. They may address issues or suggest adjustments that could make participation more manageable for you.
2. Complete an Exit Visit: The study team will likely request that you complete an "early termination" visit. This visit often includes returning unused medication, undergoing safety checks, or providing feedback about your trial experience. These steps are essential for ensuring your well-being and maintaining the integrity of the study's data.
3. Understand Potential Implications: If you withdraw mid-trial, you may forfeit certain benefits, such as access to the experimental treatment after the trial in an open-label extension or long-term monitoring provided by the study team.

⚠ Never stop taking the experimental drug or halt participation without informing the study team first. Doing so could create safety risks for you and complicate the study's data, potentially affecting results for all participants.

Withdrawing from a trial can be an emotional decision, particularly if you've built relationships with the study team or other participants. It's natural to feel conflicted. Always remember: your health and well-being come first. If you're facing challenges or doubts, communicate openly with the study team. They may offer alternative solutions, like adjusting some aspects of the trial protocol to better fit your circumstances or suggesting other trials that might suit you better. Ultimately, your participation is your choice. The clinical trial process is designed to protect your rights and prioritize your safety, even if you decide the trial is no longer the right fit for you.

Chapter 5 Highlights

- The screening visit is the first step in trial participation, where eligibility is rigorously assessed. Be prepared to undergo thorough evaluations, including medical history reviews, physical exams, lab tests, and specialized assessments.
- The informed consent is a process, not just a form. Take your time to understand the trial's risks, benefits, schedule, and commitments. Use this opportunity to ask questions and ensure clarity before signing the document.
- After qualifying during the screening visit, the baseline visit sets the stage for your participation. Randomization assigns you to a treatment or control group, ensuring scientific validity.
- Trials require regular check-ins, tests, and evaluations. Familiarize yourself with the schedule and ask the study team about telemedicine or local testing options to minimize logistical challenges.

- Your responsibilities as a participant, including adhering to the trial protocol, attending scheduled visits, completing diaries, and communicating truthfully with the study team, are essential to the trial's success and your safety.
- Clinical trial participation is always voluntary, and you have the right to stop at any time, for no reason. If you withdraw early, make sure you communicate properly with the study team.

Notes

1. Center for Information and Study on Clinical Research Participation (CISCRP), 2023, *Perceptions and Insights Study*, https://www.ciscrp.org/wp-content/uploads/2023/11/2023PI_Participation-Experiences.pdf (March 25, 2025).
2. Ibid.

6

Practical and Emotional Support during the Trial

Participating in a clinical trial involves more than following a treatment protocol; it's a commitment that can impact nearly every aspect of daily life. From managing appointments and travel to handling financial considerations and emotional ups and downs, trial participation requires careful planning and support.

This chapter explores some of the practical and emotional challenges of enrolling in a trial and offers strategies to help you stay organized, manage stress, and find the support you need. Whether it's coordinating logistics, balancing personal and professional responsibilities, or leaning on loved ones, having the right tools and resources can make the experience more manageable.

Clinical trials are a partnership between participants and researchers, and while the research study team provides medical oversight, navigating the process successfully often requires a strong support network. Here, you'll find guidance on advocating for yourself, building that network, and maintaining stability throughout the trial. With the right preparation and mindset, you can confidently approach trial participation, knowing you are contributing to medical progress while prioritizing your well-being.

Financial and Medical Insurance Implications

Understanding the financial and insurance aspects of clinical trial participation is critical for avoiding unexpected burdens and ensuring smooth participation. While sponsors typically cover the costs directly associated with the experimental treatment, other costs may arise, requiring careful planning and proactive discussions.

What Costs Are Covered in a Clinical Trial?

Sponsors typically cover the costs directly related to the investigational treatment and the trial-specific assessments, but other expenses might fall on the participant or their insurance. Here's the breakdown:

- Experimental Treatment and Administration: The investigational drug, device, or therapy being tested in the trial is usually provided at no cost. This also includes administering the therapy, such as infusion procedures or injections.
- Trial-Specific Procedures: Tests or assessments performed solely for the study's purposes, like specialized imaging, lab work, or specific evaluations outlined in the trial protocol, are generally covered.

Clinical trial participants, however, may still face costs that are not covered by the sponsor. These could include:

- Standard-of-Care Procedures: These are routine medical tests or scans that you would have undergone even if not in the trial, such as regular bloodwork or imaging for disease monitoring. These are often billed to your insurance or paid out of pocket if they are not part of the clinical trial protocol.

- Travel and Meals: While some trials cover travel costs, such as airfare, mileage, or lodging for long-distance participants, others do not. Meals and incidental expenses are typically the participant's responsibility unless explicitly covered by the trial.

- Complications and Adverse Events: If a participant experiences side effects or complications that require medical attention, the sponsor may not cover the related treatment costs. Often, the responsibility falls on the participant or their insurance unless the issue is deemed a direct result of the investigational therapy, although proving this can be challenging. Imagine a participant in a Parkinson's disease trial who suffers a fall, leading to a hip fracture. Even if the participant had no history of falls, proving the experimental drug caused the incident might be challenging due to the general risk of falls in Parkinson's patients. In such cases, the trial sponsor might argue that the injury was unrelated to the therapy, leaving the participant or their insurance to bear the medical costs.

Insurance and Out-of-Pocket Costs

Insurance coverage is critical for costs not covered by the trial sponsor. Speak with your primary healthcare provider and the trial PI or research coordinator to clarify what procedures or treatments performed during the trial visits will be covered by the sponsor or billed to your insurance.

However, even with insurance coverage, incidental costs related to participating in a clinical trial can add up:

- Travel Expenses: Transportation, parking, lodging, and meals during clinical trial visits (more on travel planning later in this chapter).
- Childcare or Dependent Care: If you have dependents, you may need to get help with childcare during your trial visits.
- Lost Wages: Time off work for travel and appointments could negatively impact your income.

Many sponsors offer stipends or reimbursement for reasonable expenses. Ask the trial coordinator about available financial assistance programs.

Financial Assistance and Resources

The financial cost associated with participation in clinical trials can sometimes be onerous. Fortunately, some organizations are willing to help.

- Patient Advocacy Groups: Many organizations, such as the American Cancer Society or the National Organization for Rare Disorders (NORD), provide grants or financial aid for trial-related expenses.
- Hospitals and Hospital Foundations: Some hospitals have funds specifically for assisting clinical trial participants. For instance, Memorial Sloan Kettering Cancer Center in New York provides travel and housing assistance, partnering with nearby hotels to offer discounted rates for patients and their families, facilitating accessibility to their clinical trials. Always ask the clinical trial team to determine if these resources are available at their hospital.

- Trial-Specific Support Programs: Large sponsors may partner with travel services or offer vouchers for expenses.
- Lodging Assistance: Organizations such as the Ronald McDonald House Charities (RMHC) offer free or low-cost housing near many hospitals and clinical trial sites for families with children participating in trials. These houses are a valuable resource for pediatric clinical trial participants, helping alleviate the burden of travel and accommodation costs. If your little one is participating in a clinical trial, make sure to check this resource out.
- Foundations Supporting Travel Expenses: Some foundations cover some travel expenses for eligible clinical trial participants. For instance:
  - Alex's Lemonade Stand Foundation: Offers travel funds for children with cancer participating in clinical trials.
  - Compass to Care: Helps with travel-related expenses for families of children receiving cancer treatment.
  - Brave and Bold Kids Foundation: Supports extended stays for families needing proximity to specialized care facilities.

Are Clinical Trial Costs Tax Deductible?

In the United States, some clinical trial-related expenses, such as travel for medical care, may be considered tax deductible as part of qualified medical expenses. However, there are specific criteria and limitations.

As of 2025, you can claim an itemized deduction for medical expenses that exceed 7.5 percent of your adjusted gross income (AGI). Travel expenses related to medical care, such as mileage, parking, and even airfare or lodging (if traveling for medical care far from home), can count toward this deduction if they are directly related to medical treatments or participation in clinical trials. Therefore, qualified travel costs while participating in the trial, such as transportation to and from the trial site and necessary lodging during the trial, may also be deductible following the above criteria. Meals are generally not deductible unless they are part of inpatient hospital care. To claim these deductions, you need detailed records of expenses, including receipts, mileage logs, and documentation showing the medical necessity of your travel or participation in the trial.

A tax advisor can help determine eligibility based on your specific circumstances. For example, if a participant travels across state lines to attend a clinical trial requiring frequent visits, the transportation costs (such as gas or public transit) and lodging could potentially be deducted, provided they meet the AGI threshold and are properly documented. Always keep detailed records of expenses and consult a tax advisor to determine if you qualify.

Navigating These Costs

To avoid surprises, ensure that you and your caregiver understand the potential financial implications by asking the trial team before enrolling in a clinical trial:

- What costs are covered by the sponsor, and what costs will be billed to my insurance?
- Will I need pre-authorization from my insurer for standard care procedures?
- Are travel stipends or other reimbursements available?
- What happens if I face unexpected costs during the trial?

Review the ICF with special attention to the cost section, as it should specify what the sponsor will and will not cover.

Check with your insurance company and ensure your current plan covers any routine care costs and potential complications that may arise during the trial participation.

⚠ Not all clinical trials are financially equal. Some trials may have generous travel stipends and additional compensation, whereas others may not. Also, be wary of trials that seem to pass too many expenses onto participants or their medical insurance without transparent communication.

With a clear understanding of financial and insurance considerations, you can better prepare for trial participation without the added stress of unexpected costs.

Travel and Logistics Planning

Participating in a clinical trial often involves more than just showing up at the trial site. Depending on the location of the study site and the frequency of visits, travel and logistical planning can become a significant part of the process. Here's how to navigate this aspect effectively and ensure smooth participation.

Choosing a Trial Site

If the trial has multiple sites, try to select the one that minimizes your travel burden. Consider factors such as:

- Proximity to Home: A nearby site reduces travel time and associated costs.
- Site Availability: Some sites may have shorter wait times or better resources.
- Trial Phases: Early phases (Phase 1 or some Phase 2) often involve more intensive monitoring and frequent visits,

making proximity even more critical. As discussed in previous chapters, I strongly advise most people against traveling for Phase 1 trials.

Plan for Travel and Accommodation

When the trial site is not local, planning is crucial:

- Transportation: When driving, factor in fuel costs, tolls, and parking availability. If you need to fly, compare costs and book tickets well in advance. Some trials may reimburse travel expenses, so confirm this with the study team.
- Lodging: If overnight stays are necessary, ask the study team for recommendations. Some sponsors partner with nearby hotels to offer discounted rates or fully cover accommodation costs. Explore extended-stay hotels or vacation rentals if the trial involves prolonged visits. In fact, some clinical trial sites collaborate with Airbnb or similar platforms to provide discounted long-term rental accommodations for families. Always ask the study team for lodging resources.

Managing Time Commitments

Balancing trial visits with work, family, and personal commitments requires careful scheduling:

- Appointment Scheduling: Coordinate appointments to minimize disruption. Early morning or late afternoon slots may be more convenient.
- Telemedicine Options: Increasingly, trials incorporate telemedicine visits for certain assessments, reducing the

need for travel. Confirm with the study team if this option is available.
- Plan for Emergencies: Keep a flexible schedule to accommodate unexpected delays or additional visits.

Budgeting for Travel

Travel costs can add up quickly. Here's how to prepare financially:

- Expense Tracking: Keep detailed records of all travel-related expenses, including transportation, lodging, and meals. As discussed above, some of these may be reimbursable or tax-deductible (always consult with a tax advisor).
- Reimbursement Policies: Check with the study team about what expenses the sponsor will cover. For instance, some trials may reimburse mileage, airfare, or hotel stays.

Some hospitals or organizations provide free or affordable transportation for medical visits, such as the American Cancer Society's Road to Recovery program. In New York City, the "Access-a-Ride Paratransit Service" provides public transportation for people with disabilities or health conditions. Check if similar services are available at your location.

Traveling with Somebody

It is always a good idea to enlist help when traveling for a clinical trial. Indeed, some clinical trials, like many for Alzheimer's disease, require that one, and sometimes two, caregivers accompany the clinical trial participant. Consider bringing, at least, one caregiver, friend, or family member as a travel companion if needed, especially for complex or physically demanding visits.

If your trial site is a long drive away, consider teaming up with another participant. If you can align your study visits, carpooling can cut costs, ease the travel burden, and even provide emotional support, turning a logistical challenge into an opportunity for connection.

🔍 Travis and James had never met before, but they were both enrolled in the same clinical trial, one I was overseeing as the PI. One day, they coincided in the waiting room, struck up a conversation, and quickly realized they had a shared challenge: traveling from each of their hometowns in Long Island, just five miles apart, to the study site in New York City and back, every two weeks. The two-hour drive was tedious and exhausting. They saw a potential solution: if their trial visits could be scheduled for the same day, they could carpool. They asked me if it was possible. Fortunately, the trial protocol allowed some flexibility, and we arranged their appointments accordingly. By taking turns behind the wheel, they not only cut their gas expenses in half but also discovered an unexpected source of strength in each other. Their biweekly drives became more than just a way to get to the trial; they became a lifeline. They swapped strategies for managing stressful moments, shared small victories, and even found humor in the quirks of trial participation. "Clinical trials can feel like a lonely road," James later told me, "but having a travel buddy changed everything. It wasn't just about saving money; it was about knowing someone else truly understood what I was going through."

Travel and logistics planning may feel daunting, but with a proactive approach, you can reduce stress and financial strain. Communicate openly with the study team about your needs and limitations; they are often willing to help find solutions that ensure your participation is as seamless as possible.

Balancing Work, Family, and Trial Commitments

Participating in a clinical trial can be demanding, particularly if you're juggling professional responsibilities, family obligations, and the trial's requirements. Striking a balance is essential to ensure your well-being and that of those around you.

Managing Work Commitments

Participating in a clinical trial may require time away from work for appointments, treatments, and recovery from potential side effects.

Since you're receiving a medical treatment or procedure requiring periodic absences, you could consider informing your manager or HR department about your participation in the trial if you're comfortable doing so. Sometimes, it can be useful to be transparent to justify your need for flexibility. However, you don't have to disclose specific medical details unless you choose.

You could request remote work or flexible hours if your job allows and use paid leave, unpaid leave, or sick days strategically for appointments and recovery.

In the United States, the Family and Medical Leave Act (FMLA) allows eligible employees to take unpaid leave for serious health conditions. Check if you qualify.

Maintaining Family Harmony

Family dynamics can be impacted by the time and energy required for trial participation. In most cases, it is a good idea to involve your family and make plans with them.

Explain the trial's importance and the potential benefits and challenges. If needed, you could share your clinical trial schedule so family members know when you'll need extra support.

If you need to delegate responsibilities, consider asking for help with household chores, childcare, or caregiving duties. Depending on where you live, you may have access to community resources, such as meal delivery services or childcare programs, to ease the burden.

It is also important to schedule some quality time. Dedicate time to connect with your family outside of the trial commitments, whether through shared meals, outings, or simple conversations.

Prioritizing Your Health

Balancing multiple commitments is only sustainable if you prioritize your well-being.

Make sure that you take your time to rest and recover. Trial participation, particularly in trials involving experimental drugs, can be physically exhausting. Listen to your body and rest as needed.

Maintain a routine, and, if possible, stick to regular meals, exercise, and sleep schedules to maintain stability.

Clinical trials can be emotionally challenging. Don't hesitate to seek counseling or therapy if needed. Check if your employer offers programs for counseling or mental health resources.

Balancing work, family, and clinical trial commitments requires open communication, strategic planning, and a willingness to seek and accept help. Remember, participating in a trial is a choice that benefits both you and medical research. By managing your commitments effectively, you can ensure a smoother journey for yourself and those who support you.

How Caregivers Can Support Trial Participants

Caregivers play a pivotal role in helping clinical trial participants manage logistics, adhere to protocols, and cope with the emotional demands of the process. Their support can make trial participation smoother and less overwhelming.

Understanding the Caregiver's Role

Caregivers are far more than passive supporters; they are organizers, companions, and advocates, playing a crucial role in ensuring that clinical trial participants can navigate the process smoothly. Whether a spouse, family member, or close friend, a caregiver's involvement can make a significant difference in the participant's ability to adhere to trial requirements and manage the physical and emotional demands of the study.

One of the caregiver's primary responsibilities is logistical support. Clinical trials often involve frequent appointments, tests, and treatments, all of which require careful coordination. Caregivers can assist by managing schedules, setting reminders for medication administration and lab visits, and ensuring that appointments aren't missed. When travel is required, they may also help arrange transportation, book accommodations, and organize itineraries to minimize logistical stress. In addition to scheduling, caregivers play an essential role in helping participants adhere to trial protocols, whether by assisting with complex dosing regimens, meal restrictions, or special preparation requirements before procedures. They also serve as an extra set of eyes, monitoring for side effects and documenting any symptoms for accurate reporting to the research team. Keeping track of essential documents, such as ICFs, study schedules, and contact information for trial coordinators, is another crucial aspect of their role.

Beyond logistics, caregivers provide emotional support, which is just as vital. Participating in a clinical trial can be emotionally demanding, leading to moments of uncertainty, anxiety, or frustration. A caregiver's presence offers reassurance, encouragement, and a compassionate space for the participant to express concerns. They provide perspective, helping to balance optimism with a realistic understanding of the experimental nature of the trial. Small acts, like celebrating milestones, whether completing a difficult visit or staying committed to a treatment plan, can make a significant impact. Understanding that mood changes are common, and that fatigue or stress can take a toll, caregivers offer companionship and steady encouragement, even in the most challenging moments.

Caregivers also serve as advocates, ensuring the participant's voice is heard and their concerns addressed. Attending appointments when possible allows them to ask questions, clarify procedures, and absorb critical information that the participant might overlook due to stress or cognitive fatigue. They help communicate any concerns to the study team, whether about unexpected side effects, logistical barriers, or the need for additional support. If adjustments are needed, such as medication modifications or scheduling changes, caregivers play a crucial role in ensuring the participant receives the accommodations necessary to continue in the trial safely.

In some trials, caregivers are also asked to complete quality-of-life or caregiver burden questionnaires. These assessments help researchers understand whether the experimental drug's effects extend beyond the participant, improving not only their health but also reducing strain on caregivers. In this way, caregivers are not only supporters but also active contributors to the trial's broader impact.

While often unseen, caregivers are the backbone of many clinical trial journeys. Their role extends beyond logistics into advocacy, emotional resilience, and ensuring that the participant's experience is as manageable, and meaningful, as possible.

For Caregivers: Balancing Responsibilities with Self-Care

Balancing the responsibilities of caregiving with self-care is essential to prevent burnout and ensure sustainable support for the participant. Caregiving can be quite taxing, and without proper self-care, the stress can take a toll on both the caregiver's well-being and their ability to provide effective support.

Recognizing personal limits is the first step. It's easy to feel obligated to handle everything alone, but overextending yourself can lead to exhaustion and frustration. Setting boundaries is crucial: defining clear limits on your availability, asking other family members to share responsibilities, or acknowledging when professional assistance is needed. Delegating tasks, even small ones, can help lighten the load and create a more manageable routine.

Seeking support is just as important as offering it. Connecting with others who understand the challenges of caregiving can provide both emotional relief and practical advice. Joining caregiver support groups, whether in person or online, allows for shared experiences, validation, and problem-solving strategies. Many caregivers find that simply talking with someone who "gets it" can ease stress and foster a sense of community.

Prioritizing personal well-being also means making time to recharge. Caregiving can become all consuming, and taking breaks, both short and extended, is necessary for maintaining mental and physical health. Scheduling moments for relaxation, hobbies, or simply stepping away from responsibilities is not a luxury but a necessity. Even small acts of self-care, like going for a walk, reading a book, or practicing mindfulness, can help restore energy and improve resilience.

Caring for someone else should not come at the expense of your health. By balancing responsibilities with self-care, caregivers can ensure that they remain emotionally and physically well enough to continue providing the support their loved ones need.

🔍 When Rose was diagnosed with metastatic breast cancer at forty-two, she and her husband, Mark, decided to participate in a Phase 2 clinical trial. As her caregiver, Mark became the steady force behind her journey, managing her medications, coordinating their out-of-town trips for treatments, and ensuring that she never faced a single appointment alone. But Mark knew that caregiving wasn't just about logistics; it was about lifting her spirit through the exhausting months ahead. After each treatment cycle, he found small yet meaningful ways to celebrate her strength, whether by arranging cozy movie nights, surprising her with handwritten notes, or bringing home her favorite French macarons. "Each milestone, no matter how small, is a perfectly good reason to celebrate," he told her. And so, with every infusion, every long drive, and every setback, Mark reminded Rose that she wasn't just a patient in a trial; she was loved, cherished, and never alone.

Caregivers are indispensable allies in the clinical trial journey. By providing practical assistance, emotional encouragement, and advocacy, caregivers ensure participants can engage with the trial while maintaining their quality of life. Equally important is for caregivers to seek their own support, recognizing that their well-being is vital to sustaining the care they provide.

Building a Support Network

In some cases, you may not need much support, especially if you're a healthy volunteer in a Phase 1 trial or participating in a low-complexity study for a nonserious condition.

However, for more demanding trials, particularly if you don't have a dedicated caregiver, a strong support network, whether through family, friends, advocacy groups, or your primary healthcare provider, can be invaluable. The right support system can help you manage logistical challenges, provide emotional encouragement, and offer a sense of community throughout your clinical trial journey. Here's how to build and maintain that network effectively.

Start with Your Inner Circle

Your family and close friends are often the first line of support during a clinical trial, but they may not fully grasp the logistical and emotional demands of participation. Be open about your needs, whether it's help with household tasks, childcare, or transportation to appointments. Sometimes, people want to assist but aren't sure how, so giving them clear suggestions (or even tasks!) to support you can make all the difference.

If you're comfortable, share your feelings and experiences with loved ones. Simply talking about your concerns or frustrations could help alleviate stress and foster a sense of connection.

💡 Pro Tip: Managing updates and coordinating support during a clinical trial can be overwhelming, especially when you're repeating the same information to different people. Free messaging apps like WhatsApp can be a game-changer. Create a group chat with family and friends so you can easily share updates, coordinate logistics, or ask for help when needed. Whether it's arranging a ride, keeping loved ones informed, or simply receiving a few words of encouragement on tough days, having a dedicated group for communication can ease the emotional burden and remind you that you're not in this alone.

Engage with the Study Team

The PI and study coordinators, as well as other clinical trial staff, are crucial parts of your network. They are trained to address your concerns, clarify questions, and provide guidance throughout the trial. Establishing a good relationship with them can make a significant difference.

Some institutions provide "patient navigators" who specialize in helping trial participants manage logistics, access resources, and connect with additional support systems. Ask if this is available at your clinical trial site.

Finding Support in Others: Online and In-Person Communities and Fellow Participants

Many trial participants turn to online communities on platforms like Facebook, Reddit, or condition-specific forums to connect with others in similar situations. These groups can sometimes offer emotional support, shared experiences, and practical advice.

In addition, hospitals, advocacy organizations, and patient support groups often host local or virtual meetings where you can discuss challenges, exchange insights, and build friendships. While these groups can be invaluable, it's crucial to remain cautious and discerning.

⚠ Be mindful of privacy. Never share personal identifying details or trial-related information that could compromise the study's integrity.

⚠ Take others' experiences with a grain of salt. No two patients or trials are identical. Just because someone claims to have had a terrible experience in a different trial, that doesn't mean their situation applies to you. Conversely, beware of the "grass is always greener" syndrome. It's natural to feel tempted when someone claims they are in a "better" trial or getting better results. However, ask yourself if they might be receiving a placebo. Moreover, switching trials isn't always possible, and dropping out of one study to chase another could mean losing access to potential treatment options. Before making any changes, revisit why you chose your trial in the first place and consult your medical team.

If your trial allows interaction, forming relationships with fellow participants could provide mutual support, companionship, and logistical benefits. As we saw before, some participants can coordinate transportation to appointments to reduce costs and stress. However, it's important to be mindful of maintaining the study integrity and confidentiality.

⚠ Never discuss specific clinical trial details. Conversations about your dose, whether you believe you're on the real drug or placebo, comparing side effects, or speculating about study results could unintentionally bias participants and skew outcomes. Discussing your feelings and challenges, celebrating milestones, or sharing what has made your journey easier with others is perfectly fine, though.

⚠ While peer support can be emotionally beneficial, it should not replace guidance from your primary healthcare or clinical trial team. Whether online or in person, the best approach is to listen, learn, and engage, but always make healthcare decisions based on your unique situation and professional advice.

Leverage Advocacy Organizations

Many condition-specific organizations, such as the Alzheimer's Association or the American Cancer Society, provide resources and connections for trial participants:

- Support Services: Some organizations offer free counseling, travel assistance, or educational materials.
- Community Events: Attend webinars, conferences, or local meetups to connect with others in similar situations.

Consider Professional Help

If managing your anxiety or addressing your feelings of disappointment or uncertainty is becoming difficult on your own, a licensed mental health professional could help you process the emotional complexities that can arise during trial participation. Look for therapists who have experience in chronic illness or medical trauma if these issues are relevant to you.

If clinical trial participation strains your budget, consulting a financial advisor could help you plan and identify economic resources, as well as determine if your expenses can be tax deductible.

Stay Open to Expanding Your Network

Your needs may evolve throughout the trial, and so should your support network. Stay open to connecting with new people or organizations that align with your current challenges and goals. You can reach out to patient advocacy groups or nonprofits for ongoing support.

Building a robust support network is not just about managing practical challenges but also about nurturing your emotional well-being. Surrounding yourself with compassionate individuals who understand your journey can make the clinical trial process more manageable and rewarding. Remember, reaching out for help is a sign of strength, not weakness. You're contributing to advancing science, but you don't have to do it in solitude.

What to Do When Things Go Wrong

Clinical trials operate under multiple layers of safety and oversight, including study coordinators, the PI, IRBs, trial sponsors, and regulatory agencies like the FDA. This system of checks and balances is designed to uphold ethical and scientific integrity.

However, despite these safeguards, deviations can still occur, ranging from minor procedural errors to serious ethical violations. Most deviations are minor and administrative, such as unaccounted-for medication doses or enrollment of a participant who slightly exceeds age limits. These typically result in correction plans issued by the IRB or study sponsor. The FDA audits clinical trial sites regularly, with most investigations addressing these minor issues. More serious violations, such as falsifying data or failing to report **serious adverse events**, are less frequent and can have far-reaching consequences. In these cases, the FDA may

- suspend or terminate the trial,
- issue warning letters requiring immediate corrective action, or
- temporarily or permanently disqualify investigators from conducting future trials.

If you believe your safety or ethical treatment has been compromised during a trial, take the following steps:

1. Review Your ICF: The ICF outlines the trial's risks, safety measures, and participant rights. It also includes the contact

information for the IRB or patient advocate associated with the trial.

2 Contact the IRB: Raise your concerns with the IRB. The IRB is legally obligated to investigate and take corrective action if necessary.

3 Reach Out to the FDA or OHRP: If the IRB fails to address your concerns satisfactorily, you can file a complaint with the FDA (FDA MedWatch) or the Office for Human Research Protections (OHRP). The OHRP focuses specifically on issues related to federally funded trials.

4 Contact the Sponsor: Most pharmaceutical companies have hotlines or email addresses for patient concerns. Communicating directly with the sponsor can sometimes expedite resolution.

🔍 In 2001, the OHRP took the extraordinary step of suspending all federally funded human research studies at Johns Hopkins University, one of the nation's premier research institutions, following the tragic death of Ellen Roche, a twenty-four-year-old healthy volunteer in an asthma study. Roche had inhaled hexamethonium, a compound not FDA-approved for human use and known to have toxic effects on the lungs. Within days, Roche suffered severe respiratory distress, ultimately leading to lung and multi-organ failure. The informed consent process failed to communicate adequately the risks associated with the experimental compound. The OHRP investigation revealed critical lapses, including the study team's failure to perform thorough literature reviews, inadequate disclosure of the experimental nature and risks of the compound, and the IRB approval of the study without fully scrutinizing its safety. The OHRP imposed a sweeping suspension across the entire institution. Johns Hopkins was required to implement significant reforms before resuming federally funded research.

This incident underscored the essential need for rigor and transparency in clinical trial oversight to protect participants and maintain public trust.

⚠ You always have the right to withdraw from any research study, including clinical trials, at any time without penalty.

⚠ You always have the right to report unethical behavior or safety violations without fear of retaliation.

Chapter 6 Highlights

- Clinical trials often cover the cost of experimental treatments and trial-specific procedures but may leave participants responsible for paying for travel, standard care, or complications.
- Plan for travel and lodging, take advantage of trial-sponsored reimbursements, and determine if you qualify for charity accommodations.
- Effectively juggle work, family, and trial demands by communicating openly with employers, delegating responsibilities, and leveraging support systems.
- Caregivers are essential for logistical, physical, and emotional support during trials.
- Encouraging self-care and building their own support networks enables caregivers to remain strong advocates for the participant.
- Trials can bring emotional highs and lows; maintaining realistic expectations and seeking emotional support can make the journey smoother.

- A robust support network of family, friends, healthcare professionals, and advocacy groups provides a critical foundation for navigating the trial process with resilience and confidence.

7

After the Trial: What Comes Next?

You are nearing the end of your clinical trial journey, or perhaps you've just completed it. Reaching this stage is momentous, not only for you but also for the advancement of science and the hope it brings to others with your condition. But now that this chapter is closing, you might be asking, what comes next?

The end of a clinical trial is often a moment of mixed emotions. For some, it brings relief, knowing that the rigorous and perhaps exhausting litany of visits, tests, and treatments is over. For others, it could stir feelings of uncertainty, especially if the investigational therapy seemed to be working for them or if it brought some hope during a challenging time. However, the end of a trial isn't an ending per se; it's a turning point.

This chapter is here to guide you through this critical transition. We'll start by breaking down the "end-of-study" visit, a crucial final step where researchers gather the last pieces of data and ensure your health and safety as you transition out of the trial. From there, we'll explore what options might be available to you, such as open-label extensions that allow you to continue receiving the experimental trial therapy or alternative paths if this isn't an option.

We'll also tackle the important topic of trial results, including how to access them, what to expect, and how to interpret unexpected findings. For many participants, understanding how the trial's outcomes fit into their broader healthcare plan is essential, whether the experimental treatment becomes a viable option for ongoing care or if adjustments need to be made. Finally, we'll touch on the emotional and practical support you might need as you navigate life after the trial.

This chapter isn't just about tying up loose ends; it's about empowering you to take the next steps with clarity and confidence, knowing that your participation has contributed to something much larger than yourself. Let's begin by exploring what happens during your final visit as a clinical trial participant.

What Happens at the End-of-Study Visit?

The "end-of-study" visit (sometimes just called the final visit) is a key milestone in the clinical trial process. This visit is designed to ensure that your health is carefully monitored as the trial concludes and to gather the final data required to evaluate the investigational treatment.

During this visit, the study team will likely perform a comprehensive set of assessments like those conducted during the screening and baseline visits. These may include

- a detailed physical exam to evaluate your current health status;
- lab tests or imaging studies to measure the impact of the experimental treatment on key biomarkers or disease progression; and
- questionnaires to assess your quality of life, symptom changes, or overall experience during the trial.

The study team will likely ask you to return any unused portions of the trial drug at your end-of-study visit. This ensures accurate inventory tracking and compliance with regulatory standards. Additionally, they will discuss the safest way to discontinue the treatment, if applicable. For some investigational drugs, abrupt discontinuation might pose risks such as withdrawal symptoms or a rebound effect, where the condition worsens temporarily. In such cases, the team will guide you through a tapering schedule or provide recommendations for follow-up care to monitor your health during this transition.

In many clinical trials, the trial medication is stopped before the end-of-study visit, often during a designated visit. After this, participants are monitored through additional follow-up visits to assess any long-term effects or delayed reactions. If this is the case, the end-of-study visit marks the final step in this monitoring phase, serving as a closure point for the trial and confirming that all required data has been collected.

This final visit is not just procedural; it's an opportunity for the study team to ensure that you are transitioning safely out of the trial. Whether the experimental treatment had a significant impact or not, their priority remains your well-being and making sure you have the information and resources needed for the next steps in your care. The study team may also provide instructions for follow-up care, including monitoring for delayed side effects after the clinical trial or addressing any lingering concerns. They might recommend additional healthcare appointments, such as follow-ups with your primary physician or specialists, based on findings during the trial. For many participants, this visit is also an opportunity to ask questions:

- When will the trial results be available?
- Will I have access to my data or learn about the treatment's outcomes?

- What are my options for continuing the treatment if I find it beneficial?

The end-of-study visit also marks the conclusion of your formal involvement in the trial. However, your relationship with the study team doesn't necessarily end here. Depending on the trial protocol, you may receive periodic updates about the study's progress, long-term results, or further opportunities to participate in related research.

⚠ If you experience new or worsening symptoms after completing the trial, it's essential to contact both your healthcare provider and the clinical trial team. This helps ensure that any delayed effects of the treatment (or its withdrawal) are properly documented and addressed.

The end-of-study visit is about closure, both for you as a participant and for the researchers gathering vital trial data. It is the bridge between your time in the trial and the next phase of your healthcare journey.

Open-Label Extension

📖 An **open-label extension (OLE)** study is a follow-up phase of a clinical trial in which all participants receive the investigational treatment, regardless of whether they were in the placebo or treatment group during the main trial. Unlike the original study, an OLE is not blinded, meaning both researchers and participants know they are receiving the active treatment.

The OLE thus provides additional data for researchers while potentially benefiting participants who can continue receiving the experimental therapy (or can receive it for the first time if they were originally assigned to the control or placebo group).

OLEs are more frequent after Phase 3 studies but can sometimes occur after Phase 2 and Phase 1 studies.

All the considerations, benefits, and logistics mentioned for OLEs also apply to extension studies. If you're unsure whether you are participating in an OLE or an extension study, ask the trial team for clarification so you can better understand the specifics of your treatment and study goals.

OLE studies are designed to address several goals:

- Ethical Considerations: For participants in the placebo group who had no chance to receive the experimental drug in the first place and for those who benefited from the investigational drug, an OLE can be seen as an ethical way to ensure continued access to a potentially beneficial treatment to patients in need of it.

- Long-Term Safety and Efficacy Monitoring: These extensions allow researchers to observe how the drug performs over an extended period. This is particularly valuable for treatments targeting chronic or progressive conditions, where long-term data can inform regulatory submissions and prescribing guidelines.

- Regulatory and Market Approval Support: Long-term data from OLEs can provide additional evidence for drug safety, efficacy, and tolerability, helping pharmaceutical companies meet regulatory requirements or better understand patient outcomes.

Sometimes, the OLE is referred to as an "extension study." The term reflects a slight difference in the study design: although participants receive the experimental drug without a placebo group, the exact dose they are receiving remains blinded. As a result, the study is not truly "open label." Extension studies provide an additional opportunity to gather critical data on whether the experimental treatment has dose-dependent effects on efficacy, biomarkers, or safety and tolerability. Importantly, like the OLE, extension studies do not include a placebo group, offering all eligible participants access to the experimental drug.

If your trial offers an OLE (or extension study), the study team should provide detailed information about the eligibility requirements, procedures, and timeline for enrollment. Here's what typically happens.

OLE Eligibility

Usually, the main requirement to participate in an OLE is to complete the main part of the trial.

⚠ If you withdrew from the trial, whether due to personal reasons, side effects, or no reason at all, you will not be eligible to participate in the OLE. This can feel disappointing, especially if you were hoping to try the experimental drug instead of a placebo. However, the exclusion is often necessary to maintain the scientific integrity of the study and ensure consistency in the data collected. It's important to remember that your decision to withdraw from a trial is always respected, and the study team should guide you toward other potential options for treatment or support. If you have questions about eligibility or alternatives, don't hesitate to reach out to the trial investigators for clarification and advice.

Many OLE studies may have specific eligibility criteria to ensure continued safety. For instance, if your status has worsened or your disease has progressed significantly, the study physician may consider that participating in the OLE may not be a good idea.

OLE Informed Consent

The OLE is often structured as a separate study. As a result, you will need to go through the informed consent process again and sign a new ICF. This document outlines the specific risks, benefits, and expectations for the OLE.

While much of the information may feel familiar, especially if the OLE closely mirrors the earlier trial, it is important to review this new ICF carefully. OLE studies may involve changes in procedures, dosing, visit schedules, or even additional risks or side effects that emerged during the initial trial. For example, the experimental drug may now be administered at a higher dose, or new data might suggest different potential side effects that require additional monitoring.

Signing the ICF confirms that you understand and accept the conditions of the OLE. It also reflects that you are providing voluntary consent to continue participating under the updated framework of the study. Make sure to ask the study team any new questions or clarify any lingering doubts about the drug, the protocol, or the follow-up plans before signing.

Remember, your participation in the OLE study, like the original trial, is entirely voluntary. Take time to review the document, discuss it with your loved ones if needed, and ensure that you are fully informed before proceeding. The study team is there to support you and address your concerns throughout the process.

OLE Assessments and Duration

During the OLE, you'll likely undergo many of the same assessments as in the original trial, such as regular lab tests, physical exams, and questionnaires. The frequency and scope of these visits may be reduced compared to the initial study, but data collection remains critical.

OLEs can last anywhere from a few months to several years. Their length often hinges on several factors, including the drug's progress toward regulatory approval, the availability of funding, and ongoing assessments of safety and efficacy. In some cases, the duration of the OLE may be extended if researchers or sponsors determine that continued access to the investigational drug benefits participants or provides additional valuable data.

Conversely, OLEs may be discontinued for various reasons. For example, if the main trial concludes that the experimental drug is ineffective, continuing the OLE would be scientifically and ethically unjustifiable. In such cases, participants are informed promptly, and the study team works with them to ensure a safe discontinuation of the investigational therapy.

OLE Cost

Typically, sponsors cover the cost of the investigational drug and study-related procedures during the OLE, just as they do in the initial trial. However, ancillary costs such as travel and routine medical care may not be covered. Always confirm what costs you might be responsible for before enrolling.

Pros and Cons of OLE Participation

For those participants who are eligible, joining an OLE offers three main advantages:

- Access to the Experimental Treatment: The OLE ensures continued access to participants originally assigned to the experimental treatment group and provides it for the first time to those who were originally assigned to the control or placebo group. Every OLE participant will get the experimental drug.

- Peace of Mind: Knowing you are receiving the active treatment, and not a placebo, can alleviate uncertainty and provide some emotional comfort.
- Additional Monitoring: Continued medical oversight during the OLE ensures that your health remains a priority.

Despite these important benefits, joining an OLE also comes with potential downsides that you should carefully consider before joining:

- Enrollment in an OLE does not guarantee that the drug will continue to be available in the future or that it will receive regulatory approval. As explained above, an OLE may be discontinued for many reasons.
- Participating in an OLE requires ongoing visits, tests, and compliance with the study protocol, which could be demanding for some participants.
- Enrollment in an OLE does not guarantee that the experimental drug provides a meaningful benefit. Sometimes, OLEs become available before there is a clear understanding of whether the experimental drug results in a clear, meaningful advantage over the control group or placebo.
- Long-term use of an experimental drug may carry unforeseen safety or tolerability risks, particularly if the drug is new or its mechanism of action is not fully understood.

An OLE can be a valuable opportunity for participants to continue receiving an experimental drug while contributing to long-term research. If offered, weigh the potential advantages and challenges carefully. Consult with your study team and primary physician to ensure that continued participation aligns with your health goals and personal circumstances.

What If an Open-Label Extension Is Not Available?

The lack of an OLE study could feel disheartening, particularly if the experimental treatment seemed promising or if you were eager to continue receiving the therapy. Several reasons may explain why an OLE is unavailable for a particular trial:

- Early Clinical Trial Stage: Most Phase 1 trials, and some Phase 2 trials, may not have an OLE, as the data on the safety and efficacy of the experimental therapy may still be incomplete and, therefore, the benefit-risk ratio of an OLE might be unclear. In these cases, sponsors may decide to wait until later clinical trial phases to offer an OLE.

- Trial Results: If the controlled portion of the trial suggests that the experimental treatment is not effective or safe, the sponsor may decide against offering an OLE. Continuing the drug under such circumstances would be unethical!

- Regulatory or Financial Limitations: The cost of providing an experimental drug to all participants without a placebo group can be prohibitive for some small pharmaceutical and biotechnological companies. Additionally, sponsors may not have the regulatory approval or resources to support a lengthy OLE.

- Transition to Market Approval: If the drug is approaching FDA approval, sponsors might prioritize moving it through the approval process over continuing trials.

While this scenario may leave you with questions and uncertainty, there are alternative avenues to explore and practical steps to take.

If an OLE study is not available, you could consider the following pathways:

- Discuss the Trial Results with Your Doctor: The PI or your primary physician can help you understand what the trial's findings mean for your condition and treatment options. If the experimental drug showed promise, your physician could monitor its progress through the regulatory process or explore similar treatments.

- Explore Expanded Access Programs (EAPs): As discussed in Chapter 3, the FDA's EAP allows patients to access investigational drugs outside of clinical trials. If the experimental therapy is no longer available through the trial but is still being studied or produced, this pathway might be an option. Work with your primary physician to determine eligibility and submit the necessary applications.

- Monitor Market Approval: If the drug has just completed all required trials and is nearing marketing approval by the FDA or other regulatory agencies, it may soon become available through traditional healthcare channels. Stay in close contact with your primary doctor and monitor pharmaceutical company announcements to learn when the drug might be accessible and covered by your medical insurance.

- Search for Other Trials: Investigate whether other trials are evaluating the same drug or similar treatments. Go back to your clinical trial spreadsheet, refine it, and consider whether joining a new trial is possible.

- Stay Involved in Advocacy: Join patient advocacy groups or organizations focused on your condition. These communities often have the latest information on treatment developments, including compassionate use programs or other patient-support initiatives.

While the absence of an OLE may seem like the end of the road, it can also mark the beginning of a new phase in your healthcare journey. By staying proactive and informed, you can explore alternative options and continue to advocate for your health and well-being.

Do Clinical Trial Participants Feel Valued?

Participating in a clinical trial is a significant commitment, one that requires time, effort, and, in many cases, personal sacrifice. Given the vital role that participants play in advancing medical research, feeling recognized and valued can make a meaningful difference in the overall trial experience.

According to the 2023 *Perceptions and Insights Study* conducted by CISCRP, among over 4,500 past clinical trial participants,[1] 86 percent of past clinical trial participants reported feeling "very" or "somewhat" appreciated during the study. However, how appreciation materialized varied widely:

- 51 percent received direct words of appreciation from the clinical trial team;
- 16 percent received a "thank you" card;
- 15 percent were invited to participate in a post-trial satisfaction survey;
- 11 percent received a small token of gratitude, such as a blanket, notebook, or water bottle;
- 5 percent received a "happy birthday" card;

- 3 percent were given a certificate recognizing their participation; and
- 32 percent, nearly one in three, received no form of acknowledgment at all.

Clinical trials rely on the generosity of volunteers who often navigate logistical challenges, time constraints, and even health uncertainties to contribute to scientific progress. A simple acknowledgment, a heartfelt thank-you, a small token, or a follow-up message can go a long way in reinforcing the value of their contribution.

If you're considering joining a clinical trial and appreciation matters to you, don't hesitate to ask the study team how they recognize participants. And if you're a researcher or trial sponsor, remember that even a small gesture of gratitude can leave a lasting impact.

Accessing Clinical Trial Data and Results

One of the most anticipated aspects of completing a clinical trial is learning the study's results and understanding what the data might mean for you and others with your condition. However, accessing data and results is not always a straightforward process. This section provides guidance on what to expect and how to navigate this phase of your clinical trial journey.

How and When Are Results Shared?

Once a clinical trial concludes, the process of analyzing and disseminating results begins. This stage involves the study sponsor conducting rigorous statistical analyses, compiling comprehensive reports, and submitting findings to regulatory agencies.

However, the timeline for public disclosure varies. While some results are released within months, others may take a year or more, depending on the complexity of the trial, regulatory requirements, and company policies.

There is no single, centralized database that contains the results of all clinical trials ever conducted (such a resource would be invaluable!).

If you're interested in accessing trial results, a simple first step is to ask the clinical study team about the expected timeline for disclosure and whether the results will be shared directly with participants. Some sponsors provide layperson-friendly summaries, but this is not always guaranteed. Being proactive and requesting this information early can improve your chances of receiving updates.

In the United States, sponsors are required to post summary results of most clinical trials on ClinicalTrials.gov within one year of the trial's completion. However, there are a few exceptions (for instance, Phase 1 trials are exempt), and not all sponsors comply with this mandate as enforcement has been inconsistent.

For publicly traded companies, it is common to release key findings through press releases on their websites. While primarily aimed at investors, these updates are publicly accessible and may provide a high-level summary of trial results.

If a trial yields significant or practice-changing results, the data may eventually be published in top medical journals, such as the *New England Journal of Medicine* (NEJM), *The Lancet*, or *Journal of the American Medical Association* (JAMA). These peer-reviewed publications offer a deeper analysis and expert commentary. However, negative or inconclusive results are less frequently published despite growing advocacy for greater transparency.

Some, though not all, trial sponsors provide participants with individual summaries revealing whether they received the active treatment or a placebo. According to the 2023 *Perceptions and Insights Study* conducted by CISCRP:[2]

- 59 percent of past clinical trial participants reported receiving a summary of the study results;
- 24 percent were informed whether they received the active treatment or placebo;
- 20 percent received information about related scientific publications;
- 19 percent received information on the brand name of the study drug (meaning, the drug had eventually received market approval); and
- 17 percent received some information on the drug approval status from the regulatory agency.

If knowing this information is important to you, ask the study team in advance whether such a summary will be provided and when you can expect to receive it.

Can You Access Your Data?

While trial results offer general insights, participants are often curious about their data. In the 2023 *Perceptions and Insights Study* conducted by CISCRP that I mentioned before, 46 percent of past clinical trial participants reported receiving some individual results, such as test results.[3] This means that, in most cases, no individual data is shared.

⚠ Accessing individual trial results is not guaranteed. Unlike routine medical tests, clinical trial results are not typically shared with participants. While regulations require aggregate clinical trial data to be made public, sponsors are not legally obligated to share individual results with participants. If knowing the individual results of the trial is important for you, proactively ask the study team about access before enrolling.

Clinical trials are designed to evaluate aggregate data, meaning your individual data is analyzed as part of a larger group. Sponsors and investigators are not typically required to share individual participant data, but some might do so if requested.

The good news is that some aspects of your trial-related data, such as lab results or imaging scans, might already be accessible to you. These are sometimes seamlessly integrated into your electronic medical records if the institution conducting the clinical trials also maintains your medical chart. For instance, if the trial involved standard bloodwork or imaging usually required for clinical care, and such tests were processed and analyzed locally at your hospital, the results might appear alongside your routine medical data in your electronic health record. If they are not readily visible in your records, you might be able to request access from the clinical trial team or the institution's medical records department. Keep in mind that more experimental or research-specific data, such as exploratory biomarkers or experimental imaging scans, may not be shared with you, as they are often part of ongoing analyses, processed by specialized vendors outside the clinical trial site or hospital, and are not validated for clinical use. In any case, feel free to inquire about what specific data you can access and how to obtain it.

If genetic testing was part of the trial, the ICF should specify whether you can access your results and at which time (before, during, or after the clinical trial). Some studies share this information with participants, especially if it has direct implications for their health or treatment, while others may temporarily or permanently withhold it due to regulatory, ethical, or study design considerations.

As discussed in Chapter 5, transparency around genetic testing results can vary, and understanding these policies upfront ensures there are no surprises later.

While transparency in clinical trials is improving, most sponsors do not provide individual results directly to participants. Sponsors are primarily obligated to regulators, not individual participants, which can leave some patients feeling disconnected from the trial's outcomes.

If you do receive some individual results (questionnaire results, laboratory test results, etc.), it's essential to interpret them in the proper context. Trial data may indicate whether the drug or therapy showed promise, had safety concerns, or failed to meet its endpoints. Discuss the results with the study physician as well as with your primary physician to understand how they might inform your ongoing care or future treatment options.

Handling Negative Clinical Trial Results

Participating in a clinical trial is a leap of faith, and it's natural to hold onto hope for positive outcomes. However, clinical trials are inherently experimental, and negative results, ranging from neutral findings to outcomes that suggest harm, are a possibility. Understanding how to navigate these scenarios with clarity and resilience is crucial for participants and their loved ones.

One of the most disheartening outcomes for participants is discovering that the experimental drug was not more effective than the placebo or control treatment. In some cases, it may even lead to worse outcomes, such as a faster progression of the disease or the emergence of unexpected adverse effects. For instance, trials in neurodegenerative diseases like Alzheimer's or Huntington's in the past have shown that some experimental drugs worsened key biomarkers and symptoms, leading to the trial's termination. These findings are not only disappointing but can feel like a personal setback, especially if hopes were high for the therapy.

If faced with such undesirable results, it's important to remember that your participation was not in vain. Trials with unexpected or negative outcomes provide critical information that shapes future research. Understanding why a drug didn't work or why it caused harm helps researchers to refine their approaches, improve safety protocols, and pave the way for more effective treatments.

When unexpected results occur, communication with the study team is vital. The trial team should share information about the findings and explain what they mean in the context of the broader research goals. If the experimental drug had adverse effects, they may recommend follow-up care or additional monitoring to address lingering health concerns. Don't hesitate to ask for a thorough explanation, as well as advice on integrating these findings into your overall healthcare plan.

Processing unexpected results can also be emotionally draining. It's normal to feel disappointment, frustration, or even grief. Acknowledge these emotions, and consider seeking support from counselors, peer groups, or organizations that specialize in your condition. Surrounding yourself with understanding and supportive individuals can help ease the burden.

Lastly, keep in mind that unexpected results do not mean the end of progress. Research is a cumulative process, and every trial, whether positive or not, adds to the collective knowledge needed to advance treatment options. By participating, you've contributed to a larger mission, one that ultimately benefits the entire patient community.

Integrating Clinical Trial Results into Your Healthcare

Participating in a clinical trial can offer valuable insights into your health and condition, which may be useful even after the study ends. However, incorporating these insights into your ongoing care requires proactive planning, coordination with your healthcare providers, and careful consideration of how the trial results fit into your overall treatment goals.

Ideally, there should be seamless communication between the clinical trial team and your primary healthcare provider, but in most cases, this doesn't happen. According to the 2023 *Perceptions and Insights Study* by CISCRP:[4]

- only 30 percent of past trial participants acknowledged the clinical trial team contacted their primary doctor for any reason;
- in 24 percent of cases, participants themselves informed their doctors about the trial results;
- in 22 percent of cases, the participant's primary healthcare provider never learned about the results; and
- only 19 percent of trial participants reported that the clinical trial team or sponsor directly shared results with their doctor.

This means that, in most cases, you are responsible for bridging the gap between the trial team and your healthcare provider. If you want your doctor to be informed, consider proactively sharing key findings and discussing how they may impact your treatment plan.

As mentioned before, you might receive information on lab tests or imaging results, mainly if they were processed locally. For example, during an experimental cancer drug trial, participants may undergo regular scans to monitor tumor size. If your imaging results show that your tumor has stabilized or shrunk, this information could guide discussions with your oncologist about whether similar drugs might benefit you or whether to maintain your current treatment approach once the trial is over. Conversely, if the scans reveal new areas of concern, your physician can evaluate whether they are related to the experimental drug or represent disease progression requiring immediate attention.

Trial-wide results, when published, can provide context for interpreting your participation and outcomes. Suppose you were part of a trial testing a new diabetes medication. The broader results might show that the drug significantly reduced blood sugar levels in participants with certain genetic markers. If you have these markers, your physician might explore approved medications that target the same pathway or consider your eligibility for follow-up trials focusing on personalized treatments.

If you are still participating in an OLE study, integrating trial results becomes even more critical. Imagine you are taking an experimental medication for rheumatoid arthritis in an OLE phase. If the trial data shows a risk of cardiovascular side effects, your doctor might recommend additional tests, such as echocardiograms, to monitor your heart health while continuing the medication. Similarly, if the OLE data suggests that higher doses yield better results, your study team and healthcare provider might discuss adjusting your dosage.

Trial results can also prompt changes to your broader healthcare strategy. For example, if a trial for an Alzheimer's treatment fails to show efficacy, your neurologist might recommend other clinical trials using experimental therapies that target different pathways.

Practical steps to integrate trial results include:

- Reviewing Trial Summaries: Ask the study team for a lay summary of the findings. For example, if a cancer trial's summary reveals that the experimental drug only benefited a subset of patients with a specific mutation, discuss with your doctor whether further genetic testing could clarify your future options.

- Discussing Results with Your Provider: Schedule a dedicated appointment to review trial outcomes and how they might influence your care. Your provider can compare trial findings with your individual results to adjust treatments or identify additional options.

- Considering Follow-Up Testing: If the trial resulted in risks, such as liver damage from an experimental drug, your doctor might recommend regular liver function tests.

- Exploring Related Trials or Treatments: Trial data might lead you to consider similar drugs or alternative trials. For instance, if a heart failure drug in a trial showed efficacy but is not yet approved, your doctor might identify a comparable approved therapy or suggest you could enroll in a clinical trial testing a similar mechanism of action.

Integrating trial results into personal healthcare is not a one-size-fits-all process. Each outcome, whether individual or trial-wide, should be interpreted in the context of your unique health journey. Open communication with your healthcare team and study staff is essential to navigate this transition effectively, empowering you to make informed decisions aligned with your health goals.

Support Systems after the Trial

🔍 After a year as a clinical trial participant for early-stage Alzheimer's, David had grown close to the study team. The routine of regular visits, cognitive assessments, and check-ins had provided a sense of stability, not just for him but for his wife, Linda, who accompanied him on every visit. When the trial ended, they expected to feel relief. Instead, Linda felt unmoored. For months, the clinical trial had been more than just medical care; it had been a lifeline. The structured visits gave her a sense of control in a situation that often felt uncontrollable. More than that, the trial team, experts in Alzheimer's, understood what she and David were going through in a way few others did. They listened, reassured her, and anticipated the challenges before she even had to ask. The PI, though not originally David's primary physician, was a renowned Alzheimer's expert. He not only guided them through the trial but also provided invaluable insights beyond the study's scope: recommendations on disease management, caregiver support, and even clinical updates that could impact David's future care. His expertise had been a compass in the storm, and now, without those check-ins, Linda wasn't sure where to turn. What made the transition even harder was that an OLE was not available. Linda had hoped that David could continue receiving the investigational treatment, but the study design didn't include this option. The abrupt stop felt like losing a safety net just when they had started to find their footing. "We walked out of those last appointments, and I felt this wave of panic," Linda recalled. "Who would I call when I had questions? Who would check on David's progress? Who would tell me what to expect next? I didn't realize how much I had relied on them, not just for David's care, but for my peace of mind." Recognizing their concerns, the study team took time to help them transition. They discussed follow-up options, connected them with local support groups, and emphasized that their journey didn't end just because the trial had. In addition, Linda asked the PI if he would consider becoming David's primary neurologist. She had come to trust his judgment deeply, and the idea of starting over with someone unfamiliar was overwhelming. To her immense relief, he agreed. This continuity provided not only expert medical guidance but also a crucial sense of stability at a time when so much else felt uncertain.

Finishing a clinical trial can be a pivotal moment in a participant's journey, bringing both a sense of accomplishment and a wave of uncertainty. The structured environment of regular visits, check-ins with the study team, and a defined treatment plan suddenly comes to an end. This transition can feel disorienting, but establishing and leaning on strong support systems (the type described in Chapter 6) can make a significant difference as you navigate the next phase.

Staying Engaged in Research

Many participants feel a sense of purpose in contributing to science and may wish to stay involved even after their trial ends. Consider exploring opportunities to participate in patient registries or biobanks, where your data can continue to contribute to research efforts. Additionally, some participants may volunteer to act as patient advocates, sharing their trial experiences at conferences, within patient communities, or during discussions with researchers and policymakers. This can be a meaningful way to remain connected to the clinical research ecosystem.

Maintaining Communication with the Clinical Trial Team

While the trial may be over, maintaining communication with the clinical trial team could still be helpful. They could provide updates on the study's progress, notify you of the publication of results, and, in some cases, inform you about open-label extensions or other trials that might interest you.

Building Long-Term Resilience

Life after a clinical trial is about integrating the experience into your broader health journey. While the trial may have answered some questions, it may also have raised new ones. Focusing on your well-being, staying informed, and remaining connected to supportive networks can help you navigate this phase with confidence and hope.

Remember, the end of a clinical trial isn't just a finish line, it's a turning point. You've gained knowledge, resilience, and insights into your health. Now, this new chapter is an opportunity to use what you've learned to make informed choices, advocate for yourself and others, and play a vital role in the advancement of medicine. Your participation has contributed to something bigger than yourself: the pursuit of better treatments, better outcomes, and hope for those who come next.

Chapter 7 Highlights

- The end-of-study visit marks the formal conclusion of your trial participation, with final tests and data collection ensuring the trial's integrity and your safety.

- An OLE may allow continued access to the experimental drug after the trial, providing valuable treatment opportunities for participants who benefited from the therapy.

- If no OLE is available, consider alternatives such as the FDA's Expanded Access Program or staying engaged with patient advocacy groups for new trial opportunities.

- Participants can access trial results through ClinicalTrials.gov, company press releases, and scientific publications. The study

team may also provide participant-friendly summaries and disclose placebo or drug assignments.
- Unexpected results, whether disappointing or surprising, require thoughtful integration into personal healthcare.
- Staying connected to a robust support system after the trial, through healthcare providers, advocacy organizations, and peer groups, helps navigate the transition and maintain continuity of care.

Notes

1. Center for Information and Study on Clinical Research Participation (CISCRP), 2023, *Perceptions and Insights Study*, https://www.ciscrp.org/wp-content/uploads/2023/11/2023PI_Participation-Experiences.pdf (March 25, 2025).
2. Ibid.
3. Ibid.
4. Ibid.

8

Addressing Unique Populations in Clinical Trials

Clinical research is not a one-size-fits-all endeavor. While most clinical trials focus on the average adult patient, certain populations, including children, individuals with rare diseases, pregnant women, and underserved communities, face unique challenges and considerations. These differences require tailored approaches to trial design, recruitment, and execution to ensure both ethical integrity and scientific validity.

Many of these groups have historically been excluded from trials due to ethical concerns, liability issues, and scientific uncertainty. For example, pregnant women are often barred from studies to avoid potential risks to the unborn child, and children were historically considered too vulnerable to participate in experimental research. However, these decisions have also left significant gaps in medical knowledge, often forcing clinicians to rely on adult data to make treatment decisions for populations with vastly different biological and physiological profiles.

Today, there is a growing recognition that including these special populations, when done ethically and rigorously, is necessary for equitable and effective medicine. Research frameworks are evolving to ensure that these populations are not just afterthoughts in clinical drug development but actively considered from the outset.

This chapter delves into the complexities of clinical trials involving these populations, beginning with pediatric research, where distinct physiological, developmental, and ethical factors guide trial design. It then explores the challenges and innovations in clinical research for pregnant women, the intricacies of rare disease trials, and the barriers faced by the elderly. Finally, it examines ongoing efforts to improve representation in trials, an essential step toward ensuring that medical breakthroughs benefit all patients.

Clinical Trials in Children

Children are not simply "small adults." Their metabolism, immune systems, and organ functions often differ significantly, which means therapies safe and effective for adults may behave differently, or fail, in pediatric populations. This demands dedicated research to ensure the safety and efficacy of treatments for younger patients. Pediatric clinical trials are a cornerstone for advancing treatments specifically tailored to children, addressing their unique physiological, developmental, and medical needs.

Despite their importance, pediatric populations remain underrepresented in medical research. Data shows a striking disparity between the number of pediatric and adult clinical trials. Only about 12 percent of trials registered on ClinicalTrials.gov focus on pediatric populations,[1] even though children bear nearly 60 percent of the disease burden for conditions studied in clinical trials.

This means that most drugs prescribed to children are evaluated only in adults. This reliance on adult data often results in **off-label prescribing**, where drugs are used in children without robust evidence for pediatric safety, dosing, or efficacy.

For instance, treatments for epilepsy, asthma, or certain cancers may require specific formulations or regimens for children. Without pediatric trials, these medications may fail to deliver optimal outcomes or pose safety risks. Similarly, diseases like certain congenital disorders or rare genetic conditions disproportionately affecting children demand specialized research that clinical trials of adult participants cannot provide.

Pediatric clinical trials are essential for defining age-appropriate dosing and developing tailored therapies for conditions unique to children, such as neuroblastoma (a pediatric cancer).

Challenges When Designing Pediatric Trials

Conducting clinical trials in children demands meticulous planning and careful consideration of their unique physiological and developmental needs. Researchers must account for the significant variability within the pediatric population, which spans from newborns to adolescents, each with distinct metabolic rates, organ functions, and developmental milestones. These differences require tailored dosing regimens and study designs to ensure both safety and efficacy. For example, a drug that is safe for a fourteen-year-old may require very different considerations for a six-month-old infant due to differences in liver enzyme activity or renal function.

Pediatric trials often prioritize endpoints that differ from adult studies, such as growth, cognitive development, or behavioral outcomes. These metrics are critical for understanding the broader impact of an experimental therapy on a child's health and development.

For example, in trials for pediatric epilepsy, researchers may assess not only a reduction in the frequency or severity of seizures but also the medication's effect on learning, memory, and overall development.

Study designs must also address the practical challenges of working with children. Many younger participants cannot communicate symptoms effectively, making it essential for trials to rely on validated caregiver-reported outcomes or objective measures. Procedures that might be routine for adults, such as blood draws or imaging, often require additional adjustments for children. For instance, acquiring a brain scan for a child may require sedation to ensure they remain still during the procedure, especially for toddlers and young children who might struggle to understand the importance of staying motionless for fifteen to twenty minutes.

Another critical aspect is the drug's **formulation** (i.e., whether it comes as a pill, capsule, or other form). Children may struggle with swallowing pills, requiring researchers to develop liquid, chewable, or dissolvable formulations. For example, the development of child-friendly liquid medications for antiretroviral therapy in HIV-infected children was a breakthrough in improving adherence and outcomes.

Ethical Considerations and Informed Consent in Pediatric Trials

Ethical considerations are at the heart of pediatric clinical trials due to the unique vulnerabilities of children as participants. Unlike adults, children cannot provide legal consent to participate in research. Instead, their parents or legal guardians must act as proxy decision makers, weighing the potential risks and benefits on behalf of their child. This process must be thorough, transparent, and sensitive to the emotional and ethical complexities involved.

Informed consent for pediatric clinical trials involves obtaining permission from the child's parent or guardian. This consent process must be comprehensive, explaining in detail the purpose of the trial, the procedures involved, the potential risks and benefits, and the alternatives to participation. Parents should feel fully informed and empowered to make decisions in the best interests of their children.

However, researchers often go a step further to involve the child in the decision-making process. For children who are old enough to understand, researchers typically seek their "assent."

📖 **Assent** is the child's voluntary agreement to participate, distinct from the legal concept of consent. It demonstrates respect for the child's developing autonomy and ensures that the child is comfortable with the decision to participate.

The process of obtaining assent varies depending on the child's age, maturity, and cognitive ability. For example, for younger children, researchers may explain the trial in simple, relatable terms, such as using drawings or stories to describe what will happen. Older children and adolescents can engage in more detailed discussions about the study, including potential risks and discomforts.

Obtaining assent often involves creative approaches to engage children in a way that respects their developmental stage. Researchers might explain blood draws to younger children as "a quick pinch to help doctors learn more about your health." For older children, researchers might provide simplified versions of the informed consent document, using visuals or videos to enhance understanding.

The child's right to **dissent** is important. Even if a parent consents, a child's refusal to participate is usually respected, especially in non-life-threatening scenarios. Researchers must strike a delicate balance between respecting the child's autonomy and addressing the family's health priorities.

Ethical guidelines require that the risks posed to pediatric participants be minimized and justified by the potential benefits to the child or the knowledge gained for the broader societal good. This principle is critical because children may not fully understand the implications of their participation. Trials involving minimal risk, such as observational studies, are generally easier to justify than those involving invasive procedures. In cases of serious illnesses, such as cancer, where standard treatments have failed, the potential benefit of accessing an experimental therapy may outweigh the risks, making participation ethically defensible.

Several safeguards ensure the ethical conduct of pediatric trials:

- Institutional Review Boards (IRBs): Before any clinical trial begins, IRBs must approve the study protocol, ensuring that risks are minimized and parental consent and child assent processes are robust.
- Pediatric Ethics Committees: Some institutions have specialized committees to review trials involving children, providing an additional layer of scrutiny.
- Federal Regulations: In the United States, the FDA and the Department of Health and Human Services enforce regulations specific to pediatric research, such as Subpart D of the Common Rule, which outlines additional protections for children as research participants.

Respecting the dignity and rights of pediatric participants and their families is essential. Trial teams must create a supportive environment where parents feel confident in their decisions and children feel heard and cared for. This approach upholds ethical standards and fosters trust, ensuring that families feel respected and valued throughout the clinical trial experience.

Questions to Ask before Enrolling Your Child in a Clinical Trial

Enrolling a child in a clinical trial is a significant decision, and parents or guardians should feel fully informed before proceeding. As a parent, your responsibility is to understand the trial's purpose, risks, and potential benefits. Often, parents hesitate due to concerns about potential risks or discomfort, while logistical issues like frequent hospital visits and time away from school can create barriers. The study team should provide comprehensive information to help you make an informed decision.

Here are key questions to ask the research team to ensure the study is safe, ethical, and the right fit for your child. While some of these questions may also apply to adult clinical trials, they are especially critical when considering a trial for a child, given the unique medical, ethical, and developmental factors involved.

- What is the purpose of this study?
- How was this trial designed for children rather than adults?
- Has this treatment been tested in other children before? If so, how many, and what were the results?
- What phase is the trial in, and what does that mean for my child's participation?
- What are the potential benefits and risks of participation?
- Were side effects identified in past trials in adults or children? If so, how will the adult doses relate to the doses studied in my child?
- How are side effects monitored, and what happens if my child experiences one?

- Are there any long-term risks?
- Who will oversee my child's safety throughout the trial?
- Who will pay for medical treatment if my child is injured or suffers an adverse event or side effect that requires treatment during the trial?
- What tests, procedures, or treatments will my child undergo?
- How often will we need to visit the study site, and how long will each visit take?
- Will my child need to stay in the hospital, miss school, or restrict daily activities?
- What are the standard treatment options outside of this trial?
- Can we withdraw from the trial at any time if we change our minds?
- Will we receive financial support for travel, lodging, or other costs?
- If my child responds well to the treatment, can they continue receiving it after the trial ends?
- Will we be informed of the trial results once it's over?
- Have any studies been conducted with this compound in juvenile mice, rats, or other animals?

After your questions have been answered, discuss the trial with your child, using age-appropriate language to explain what to expect.

It is important to know that many hospitals and organizations offer resources, including support groups and financial assistance, to help families navigate the complexities of trial participation. While we reviewed some of these resources in Chapter 6, do not hesitate to ask the clinical trial team.

Pediatric clinical trials offer hope and new possibilities for children facing medical challenges. While participation requires careful consideration, the potential benefits to the child, their peers, and future generations can be transformative.

Clinical Trials in Other Vulnerable Populations

In clinical trials, certain groups are categorized as vulnerable due to their specific needs, potential risks, and challenges in participation. Beyond children, who were discussed in the previous section, vulnerable populations typically include pregnant women, the elderly, individuals with mental illnesses, and prisoners.

Enrolling these groups in clinical research obliges additional ethical and logistical considerations to safeguard their safety and autonomy. Their inclusion is often essential to understanding how treatments work across diverse populations, yet the associated complexities often lead to their exclusion. Striking the right balance between ensuring safety and generating meaningful data is key to making clinical trials equitable and representative. Let's examine the unique considerations for each group.

Pregnant Women

Pregnant women have long been excluded from clinical trials, with only about 1 percent of trials allowing their participation.[2] This exclusion stems from well-intentioned concerns about potential harm to the unborn child from experimental drugs.

🔍 Thalidomide, introduced in the 1950s as a sedative and treatment for morning sickness, caused severe birth defects in thousands of babies. At the time, safety testing in pregnant women was minimal, and the drug's effects on fetal development went undetected during its limited trials. The tragedy prompted stricter drug approval regulations worldwide, including the requirement to test drugs in pregnant animals and conduct more extensive clinical trials. Today, the lessons learned from thalidomide guide the rigorous safety protocols designed to protect vulnerable populations, including pregnant women and their babies.

The problem is that these protective measures have unintentionally created significant gaps in understanding how medications and treatments affect pregnancy and fetal development. This lack of data poses risks for conditions like hypertension, diabetes, infections, or other illnesses requiring treatment during pregnancy. Alarmingly, up to 80 percent of pregnant women are prescribed therapies that have never been studied in clinical trials allowing the participation of pregnant women.[3]

For pregnant women to safely participate in clinical trials, the design must consider dual risks to both the mother and the unborn child. Such trials demand rigorous preclinical safety data, meticulous monitoring (including regular ultrasounds and specialized fetal assessments), and an informed consent process that transparently outlines risks to both mother and child. Regulatory agencies and institutional ethics boards impose additional layers of scrutiny on these trials to ensure that the highest standards of safety and ethics are met.

Recent developments, such as the inclusion of pregnant women in COVID-19 vaccine trials, have highlighted the importance of generating evidence-based guidelines for this population. This was an important step toward the enrollment of pregnant women in clinical trials to ensure they had access to the vaccine.

Despite growing advocacy for including pregnant women in clinical trials, significant challenges persist. This continued issue maintains critical gaps in medical knowledge, leaving questions unanswered about which medications are safe, which interventions are effective, and whether delaying treatment until after pregnancy is advisable.

Without clinical trial data on pregnant women, healthcare providers often rely on off-label prescribing or extrapolate from adult data, increasing uncertainty in treatment outcomes. As a result, pregnant women and their physicians are frequently forced to make decisions with incomplete information, potentially compromising care for both the mother and the baby, underscoring the urgent need for innovative, ethical solutions to bridge this critical gap in clinical research.

Elderly Populations

Older adults, defined as those aged sixty-five years and older, represent approximately 17 percent of the US population but account for 34 percent of all prescription medication use. Nearly 90 percent of older adults report taking at least one prescription drug.[4]

Despite their significant presence in the healthcare landscape, older adults remain underrepresented in clinical trials, particularly for treatments they are likely to receive. While trials for conditions such as Alzheimer's disease and osteoporosis, which predominantly affect older populations, often include them, only about 8 percent of clinical trials enroll individuals aged eighty and older.[5] This exclusion persists despite the unique medical challenges older adults face, including age-related physiological changes, multimorbidity (having three or more chronic conditions), and polypharmacy (taking multiple medications).

The exclusion of elderly participants from clinical trials has potentially negative implications. Age-related changes, such as slower liver and kidney metabolism, can alter how drugs are processed, affecting both efficacy and safety. Clinical trials often fail to address these variations, leaving physicians with inadequate data to guide prescribing decisions. For example, drugs that appear effective and safe in younger populations may have reduced efficacy or increased side effects in older adults. Additionally, trials rarely focus on outcomes particularly meaningful to this demographic, such as improvements in mobility, cognitive function, quality of life, or independence.

Certain barriers contribute to the underrepresentation of older adults in trials. Many studies exclude them due to concerns about frailty, comorbidities, or their inability to adhere to complex protocols. Residents of long-term care or assisted living facilities are especially marginalized. This exclusion limits the generalizability of trial results and creates a gap in understanding how treatments perform in real-world elderly populations.

Efforts to address these issues include removing unnecessary age-related eligibility criteria, reducing logistical burdens such as transportation challenges, and designing trials with more relevant endpoints. For conditions like dementia, involving caregivers in the process can help ensure informed consent and adherence to study protocols. For instance, Alzheimer's trials frequently rely on caregiver input to evaluate both safety and efficacy comprehensively.

Legislative action has also begun to address these gaps. The Consolidated Appropriations Act of 2023 includes mandates for clinical trial diversity, which applies to the inclusion of older adults. These measures are a step toward ensuring that clinical research reflects the populations most likely to use new treatments. Despite these advancements, significant work remains to create a system where older adults are adequately represented in clinical trials. By including this population, researchers can provide prescribers with the necessary data to optimize care for an aging society.

People with Mental Health Disorders

Millions of people worldwide take medications for mental health conditions, including depression, bipolar disorder, schizophrenia, and anxiety disorders. While psychiatric medications must be rigorously tested in individuals who have these conditions, conducting clinical trials for mental illness presents unique ethical, practical, and scientific challenges.

One of the primary barriers is informed consent. Clinical trials require participants to fully understand the study's risks, benefits, and procedures before enrolling. This can be complex for individuals with cognitive impairment, psychosis, or severe mood disorders that affect judgment and comprehension. As a result, most trials tend to include participants with mild to moderate psychiatric conditions, often excluding those with severe illness, which in turn limits the generalizability of research findings. In cases where a participant's decision-making capacity is impaired, a legally authorized representative (such as a guardian or close family member) may provide consent on their behalf.

Beyond informed consent, safety protocols are especially critical in psychiatric trials. Many mental health conditions come with risks such as suicidal ideation, self-harm, or unpredictable behavioral changes. Therefore, trials involving psychiatric medications require enhanced monitoring, including

- frequent mental health check-ins to assess symptom changes;
- emergency intervention plans in case a participant's condition worsens;
- carefully designed eligibility criteria to minimize risks for vulnerable participants; and

- simplified study materials and instructions to accommodate cognitive impairment, ensuring participants can adhere to protocols effectively.

For example, in clinical trials for schizophrenia medications, researchers often employ continuous psychiatric monitoring, ensuring that participants receive immediate intervention if they experience worsening symptoms, medication side effects, or heightened distress.

If you or a loved one is interested in participating in psychiatric clinical trials, the National Institute of Mental Health (NIMH), a branch of the NIH, conducts numerous studies aimed at advancing treatments for mental health disorders in both adults and children. Additionally, academic medical centers and major research institutions frequently offer clinical trial opportunities designed to improve psychiatric care.

Prisoners

Prisoners are a vulnerable group whose inclusion in clinical trials demands heightened ethical considerations. Historically, incarcerated individuals were subjected to exploitation in medical research, often without their informed consent or any regard for their welfare.

🔍 One of the most infamous cases of unethical medical research involving prisoners occurred at the Holmesburg Prison in Philadelphia between the 1950s and 1970s. Under the direction of Dr. Albert Kligman, a dermatologist from the University of Pennsylvania, inmates were subjected to a wide range of experiments involving chemical agents, pharmaceutical drugs, and even biological warfare compounds, all without true informed consent. Kligman, best known for his later development of Retin-A (tretinoin) for acne, reportedly saw the prisoners as a "captive audience" for his research. The studies, many of which were funded by the US Army, major pharmaceutical companies, and the CIA, tested substances ranging from dioxin (a toxic component of Agent Orange) to skin-burning chemicals and hallucinogens. Many prisoners suffered long-term health consequences yet were largely unaware of the risks when they agreed to participate, often in exchange for small financial incentives.

These experiments became a stark example of the ethical failures in prisoner research, eventually leading to stricter federal regulations. In 1978, the US government severely restricted the use of prisoners in medical research, recognizing their vulnerability to coercion and exploitation.

Today, research involving incarcerated individuals is tightly regulated under Subpart C of the Common Rule (45 CFR 46) to prevent abuses like those seen at Holmesburg. Researchers must eliminate any hint of coercion or undue influence, such as offering reduced sentences, improved living conditions, or other incentives that could impair free choice. Trials involving prisoners are subject to additional reviews by IRBs and must comply with specific federal regulations, which outline protections for prisoners in research.

The participation of prisoners in clinical trials should aim to improve healthcare access for a population that often experiences significant health disparities. For example, recent clinical trials investigating treatments for hepatitis C have included prison populations because of the disease's high prevalence among incarcerated individuals. These studies provided an opportunity for prisoners to access potentially lifesaving treatments while generating valuable data to address public health challenges.

Clinical Trials for Rare Diseases

Rare diseases, also referred to as orphan diseases, are defined as conditions affecting fewer than 200,000 people in the United States. Globally, there are approximately 7,000 identified rare diseases, collectively impacting an estimated 300 million individuals. Despite the small patient populations for individual diseases, rare diseases as a group affect around 5–10 percent of the global population. Most of these conditions are genetic, severe, albeit chronic, and slowly progressive, with many manifesting in childhood.

Historically, rare diseases were neglected by pharmaceutical companies due to the limited market potential and high cost of drug development. Before the 1980s, there was little incentive to invest in treatments for these conditions, leaving millions of patients without effective therapies. The landscape began to shift with the passage of the **Orphan Drug** Act (ODA) in the United States in 1983. This legislation offered incentives to companies developing treatments for rare diseases, including:

- Grants for research and development: The FDA's Orphan Products Grants Program provides funding to academic institutions, small biotech companies, and researchers developing treatments for rare diseases. These grants support preclinical studies and clinical trials.

- Tax credits covering 50 percent of clinical trial costs: Pharmaceutical companies can claim tax credits up to 50 percent of qualified clinical trial costs for orphan drug development. These costs include expenses directly related to conducting trials, such as site fees, patient recruitment, and data analysis.

- Waivers of FDA application fees: Orphan drug developers are exempt from paying the FDA's user fees, which can be substantial (e.g., over $3 million for a **new drug application** in 2023). This applies to fees for applications as well as annual establishment and product fees.

- Seven years of market exclusivity for approved orphan drugs: This means that the FDA will not approve another similar drug for the same rare disease during this period. This exclusivity applies regardless of patent status, meaning competitors cannot market a **generic** or similar drug for the same condition.

All these incentives spurred significant growth in rare disease research. Before the ODA, only thirty-eight orphan drugs had been approved. Since its enactment, more than 1,000 orphan drugs have gained FDA approval, representing approximately 35 percent of all new drug approvals in recent years.

Rare diseases account for a growing percentage of clinical trials, thanks to advances in genomics, precision medicine, and increased awareness. Estimates suggest that around 10–15 percent of clinical trials globally focus on rare diseases. In the United States, the percentage of new drug approvals for orphan indications has steadily increased, with orphan drugs making up 55 percent of new FDA-approved drugs in 2022.

Challenges in Rare Disease Trials

Conducting clinical trials for rare diseases presents unique challenges. With limited numbers of eligible patients, recruitment can be challenging. Trials often require multicenter, international collaboration to enroll enough participants. Many rare diseases have variable symptoms, complicating the establishment of clear inclusion criteria and endpoints. The lack of information about how the disease evolves (natural history) makes it difficult to define meaningful trial endpoints.

Consequently, changes in biomarkers are often used in rare disease trials because traditional clinical outcomes (e.g., survival) would require impractically long studies. Demonstrating efficacy and safety with small sample sizes requires innovative trial designs. Most importantly, patients, families, and patient advocacy groups and foundations must play an important role in trial awareness, recruitment, and participation.

To address these challenges, researchers and sponsors often adopt innovative approaches:

- Adaptive Trial Designs: The design of the trial may evolve as interim data becomes available, allowing for modifications to endpoints, duration, number of participants, or eligibility criteria.

- Use of Real-World Evidence (RWE): Data from patient registries, natural history studies, and electronic health records can supplement clinical trial findings and, sometimes, be used instead of a placebo group.

- N-of-1 designs: Sometimes, the disease is so rare that clinical trials of one participant are accepted as sufficient evidence for drug efficacy, like in Mila's case (discussed in Chapter 3).

🔍 In 2017, the FDA approved Brineura® (cerliponase alfa) for treating CLN2 disease, an ultra-rare, fatal pediatric neurodegenerative disorder. Brineura®'s approval exemplifies the challenges and innovation in developing therapies for ultra-rare conditions. The pivotal trial supporting Brineura®'s approval deviated from standard placebo-controlled designs due to ethical and logistical concerns. It was an open-label trial involving twenty-four children, where all participants received Brineura®, avoiding the ethical dilemma of withholding treatment from children with a rapidly degenerative condition. Instead of a placebo group, efficacy was evaluated using external, historical data from untreated children, focusing on changes in motor and language abilities assessed by the CLN2 clinical rating scale. The results were compelling: treated participants experienced significantly slower disease progression compared to the rapid progression of untreated children who were not part of the trial. Brineura®'s approval highlighted the importance of natural history data and innovative trial designs for ultra-rare diseases. BioMarin, the pharmaceutical company developing the drug, benefited from the incentives of the ODA.

With advances in genetic diagnostics, gene therapies, and precision medicine, the outlook for rare disease research is brighter than ever. Programs like the FDA's Rare Diseases Program and initiatives from organizations such as the EMA further support these efforts. Yet, continued advocacy, funding, and innovation are essential to ensure that every rare disease patient has a chance at effective treatment.

Increasing Representation in Clinical Trials

Representation (sometimes referred to as diversity) in clinical trials means ensuring that the population participating in a study closely mirrors the population that will ultimately use the drug in the real world. For example, if an Alzheimer's treatment is intended for both elderly men and women, clinical trials should aim to enroll participants in proportions reflective of that intended use. This principle could extend to other factors like ethnicity and geographic origin.

An FDA report analyzing data from 2015 to 2020 revealed some disparities in clinical trial representation.[6] Among more than 100,000 participants in US sites in 517 trials, 76–81 percent were White/Caucasian (aligning closely with US census data). However, Asian representation was low at just 2–3 percent, while African American/

Black participants made up 15–19 percent, exceeding their proportion in the US population. Hispanic enrollment ranged 10–20 percent, falling short of US demographics, and American Indian/Alaska Native representation was very low at just 0.6 percent.

Several factors contribute to these discrepancies. Practical barriers, such as living far from trial sites or lacking access to childcare, play a role. Personal choice is also significant, as clinical trial participation is voluntary, and individuals may opt out for various reasons. Cultural and social influences can further impact participation rates, particularly among underrepresented groups.

Addressing these challenges requires innovative approaches. One notable example is the "barbershop study," which creatively engaged African American communities to increase trial awareness and participation.

🔍 A groundbreaking study showcased a culturally tailored approach to clinical trials that significantly improved hypertension among African American men.[7] Conducted in fifty-two barbershops across Los Angeles, this open-label, controlled clinical trial enrolled 319 African American men with poorly controlled hypertension. Participants were randomized into two groups. In the first group, barbers encouraged patrons to consult with specialty-trained pharmacists who operated directly within the barbershop. These pharmacists provided antihypertensive medications, monitored blood pressure, and offered lifestyle counseling. In the second group (control group), barbers provided standard lifestyle advice and encouraged patrons to follow up with their primary physicians. After six months, the results were striking. The intervention group experienced an average blood pressure reduction of 27 mmHg compared to a modest reduction of 9.3 mmHg in the control group. Moreover, 89.4 percent of the intervention group achieved blood pressure control (i.e., they no longer had hypertension) compared to only 32.2 percent in the control group. Barbershops, trusted spaces within African American communities, provided an accessible and familiar environment, overcoming the barriers of healthcare systems. The presence of pharmacists ensured that clients received immediate, personalized care, avoiding logistical hurdles like scheduling appointments at medical offices. The study highlights the success of meeting patients where they are, both literally and culturally.

Other successful initiatives have included partnerships with community centers, religious organizations, and advocacy groups. Decentralized trials using telemedicine and local healthcare providers have minimized logistical barriers for rural and low-income participants (more on decentralized trials in the next chapter). Tailored educational campaigns, such as providing materials in Spanish and involving community leaders, have also helped engage Spanish-speaking communities more effectively.

Advocates of increasing representation argue that enrolling diverse ethnicities in clinical trials can help better understand the safety and efficacy of drugs. This is clear for Asian populations, particularly Japanese and Chinese, who often require dedicated clinical trials due to differences in genetic makeup and physiology that can significantly influence drug safety and efficacy. These tailored trials are essential to ensure that therapies are optimized for diverse populations and are not based solely on data from Western participants.

For example, differences in drug metabolism are a major factor driving the need for clinical trials in Asian populations. Genetic polymorphisms in enzymes like cytochrome P450 (CYP) are more prevalent in these groups and can dramatically alter how drugs are processed. For example, CYP2C19 variants affecting the metabolism of clopidogrel, a commonly prescribed blood thinner, are more frequent in Asians, leading to reduced drug efficacy and higher cardiovascular risks. Similarly, CYP3A5 variants influence the metabolism of immunosuppressants like tacrolimus, requiring adjusted doses for Asian transplant patients.

Other differences, such as lower average body weight and variations in fat distribution, impact how drugs are absorbed and distributed. Many drugs dosed based on body weight or surface area require testing in Asian populations to determine appropriate dosing. Environmental factors, such as diet, also play a role. High consumption of foods like green tea or soy in Asian diets can interact with drug metabolism, affecting efficacy and safety. There are also regulatory requirements. The regulatory agencies in Japan and China typically mandate local clinical trials for drug approval. This ensures that therapies are rigorously evaluated for their populations, reducing risks associated with extrapolating data from Western trials.

Genetic variations impacting the response to experimental drugs are also prevalent in other populations. For instance, CYP2D6 polymorphisms affecting antidepressant metabolism are more common in African and Middle Eastern populations.

While many argue that this is an important reason to enroll racially diverse populations, others adduce that a diverse ethnic background may not always align with a genetically diverse background. The complexity arises because ethnicity is self-reported (there are no genetic markers for ethnicity or race) and exists on a continuum, making objective categorizations difficult. This complexity requires nuanced trial designs that prioritize genetic and environmental diversity over simplistic ethnic classifications.

By addressing cultural, logistical, and systemic barriers, clinical trials can better reflect real-world populations, enhancing the development of effective medical treatments. Continued innovation and community engagement are essential to achieving this goal.

Chapter 8 Highlights

- Children's unique physiology and needs require tailored trial designs and ethical safeguards, including assent alongside parental consent.

- Groups like pregnant women, the elderly, and prisoners face distinct challenges in trials, requiring specialized protocols to ensure safety and equity.

- Innovative designs, such as natural history comparisons, address the challenges of small participant pools in clinical trials of rare diseases.

- Efforts like culturally tailored outreach and decentralized trials aim to improve the representation of underserved populations.

Notes

1   Sara K. Pasquali, Wendy K. Lam, Karen Chiswell, Alex R. Kemper, and Jennifer Li, "Status of the Pediatric Clinical Trials Enterprise: An Analysis of the US ClinicalTrials.gov Registry," *Pediatrics* 130, no. 5 (November 2012): e12679–e1277.

2   Alyssa Bilinski and Natalia Emanuel, "Fewer than 1% of United States Clinical Drug Trials Enroll Pregnant Participants," *American Journal of Obstetrics and Gynecology*, 232, no. 4 (April 2025): e136–e139.

3   Katrina Heyrana, Heather Byers, and Pamela Stratton, "Increasing Participation of Pregnant Women in Clinical Trials," *Journal of the American Medical Association* 320, no. 20 (November 18, 2018): 2077–78.

4   Janice B. Schwartz, "Representative Enrolment of Older Adults in Clinical Trials: The Time Is Now," *Lancet Healthy Longevity* 4 (July 7, 2023): E301–E303.

5   S. W. Johnny Lau, Yue Huang, Julie Hsieh, et al., "Participation of Older Adults in Clinical Trials for New Drug Applications and Biologics License Applications from 2010 through 2019," *JAMA Network Open* 5, no. 10 (October 14, 2022): e2236149.

6   Milena Lolic, Richardae Araojo, Melvyn Okeke, and Janet Woodcock, "Racial and Ethnic Representation in US Clinical Trials of New Drugs and Biologics, 2015–2019," *Journal of the American Medical Association* 326, no. 21 (December 7, 2021): 2201–3.

7   Ronald G. Victor, Kathleen Lynch, Ning Li, Ciantel Blyler, et al., "A Cluster-Randomized Trial of Blood-Pressure Reduction in Black Barbershops," *New England Journal of Medicine* 378, no. 14 (March 12, 2018): 1291–1301.

9

The Future of Clinical Trials: Innovation and Empowerment

As we stand on the cusp of a new era in clinical research, the question is no longer just how we conduct trials but how we redefine them. Emerging innovations, from decentralized trials that bring research to your doorstep to the game-changing potential of AI and wearable technologies, are reshaping how new therapies are tested and approved. Could we one day eliminate traditional clinical trials?

Yet, amid these advancements, perhaps the most profound shift is not technological; it's human. The growing recognition that patients are not just participants but partners is transforming the clinical trial landscape. No longer passive subjects following rigid protocols, they are becoming advocates, decision makers, and catalysts for change.

In this final chapter, we'll explore the future of clinical trials and the critical improvements needed to ensure that research is not only more efficient and innovative but also more patient centered. In the end, clinical trials aren't just about developing new treatments; they're about the people who make those breakthroughs possible.

How Could Drug Development and Clinical Trials Be Improved?

Drug development, in general, and clinical trials, in particular, are foundational to medical progress. However, they are often criticized for their inefficiencies, high costs, rigidity, and limited accessibility. Improving drug development and clinical trials is not just about incremental change; it requires a bold rethinking of how studies are conducted, who participates, and how data is collected and analyzed.

Could Animal Testing Be Avoided?

In the preclinical stages, some have challenged the long-standing reliance on animal studies in drug development. Technologies like "organ chips," tiny, bioengineered devices lined with human cells that mimic the behavior of specific organs, are providing new insights into how drugs interact with the body. Similarly, organoids, which are miniature, simplified versions of human organs grown from stem cells, allow researchers to study disease processes and drug effects in human-like systems. Advanced computational models powered by AI can simulate drug interactions in virtual environments, reducing the need for human participants.

In a significant regulatory shift, a 2022 law signed by President Biden allows the FDA to approve drugs based on nonanimal preclinical tests, such as the above-mentioned advanced technologies. While this marks a major step forward, animal studies remain the standard in most cases due to their ability to evaluate complex biological responses across an entire living system, something even the most advanced models cannot yet replicate. For example, testing for immune system reactions or long-term toxicity often requires the full biological interplay that only animal models can currently provide. So, while the law allows the FDA to consider nonanimal testing, it is highly unlikely that the FDA will green-light drugs that have not undergone animal testing. However, with ongoing advancements in technology, the reliance on animal studies may continue to diminish, paving the way for more precise testing methods in the future.

Improvements in Clinical Trial Recruitment, Design, and Transparency

An important area for improvement is participant recruitment and retention. Currently, over 80 percent of clinical trials face delays due to difficulty enrolling participants, and up to 30 percent of enrolled participants drop out before completing the trial. Streamlining recruitment through better outreach (using community partnerships, digital platforms, and patient advocacy groups) could help close these gaps. Similarly, reducing trial burdens like frequent travel with decentralized trials (see next section) or invasive procedures could improve retention.

The clinical trial design process also demands innovation. Traditional randomized placebo-controlled trials, often viewed as the gold standard, are sometimes too rigid for real-world applications. "Adaptive trial designs," which allow for protocol adjustments based on interim results, offer more flexible and efficient alternatives. For example, during the COVID-19 pandemic, adaptive platform trials like the RECOVERY trial in the United Kingdom enabled researchers to rapidly test multiple treatments for effectiveness in real time, saving precious time and resources.

🔍 The "Randomized Evaluation of COVID-19 Therapy" (RECOVERY) trial, launched in March 2020 in the United Kingdom, became a groundbreaking example of an adaptive platform trial, a flexible design that allows researchers to test multiple treatments simultaneously and modify protocols based on interim results. At the height of the pandemic, the trial rapidly enrolled tens of thousands of patients across hundreds of hospitals, testing a range of potential COVID-19 therapies. One of its most significant findings was that dexamethasone, a widely available corticosteroid, reduced mortality by one-third in ventilated patients and by one-fifth in those requiring oxygen, a discovery that immediately changed clinical practice worldwide. Unlike traditional randomized controlled trials, which can be slow and rigid, RECOVERY's adaptive design swiftly discontinued ineffective treatments (e.g., hydroxychloroquine and lopinavir-ritonavir) while redirecting resources toward promising therapies. This efficiency not only saved lives but also demonstrated the potential of adaptive trial methodologies in responding to public health crises.

Another critical improvement area is transparency. Clinical trial participants increasingly expect access to trial data, including results and their contributions. Expanding open-access data initiatives, such as those supported by the AllTrials campaign, can foster trust and accelerate scientific discovery.

🔍 Launched in 2013, the AllTrials campaign advocates for greater transparency in clinical research, demanding that all past and present clinical trials be registered and their full results reported. The initiative has gained support from thousands of researchers, organizations, and policymakers worldwide. Historically, a significant portion of clinical trial data, especially for unsuccessful or negative results, remained unpublished, leading to incomplete evidence for medical decision-making. AllTrials aims to close this gap by pushing for reforms that mandate trial registration, data sharing, and public availability of results. The campaign has influenced global policies, contributing to European Union clinical trial transparency laws and pressuring pharmaceutical companies and research institutions to disclose trial results. However, challenges remain, particularly in balancing data transparency with patient privacy and ensuring compliance with transparency initiatives. By promoting open-access data, the AllTrials movement fosters trust in clinical research, enables more reliable access to clinical trial data, and accelerates scientific discovery for the benefit of all patients.

Could We Perform More Clinical Trials in Low- and Middle-Income Countries?

Addressing global disparities in clinical trial access is essential. While much of the world's population resides in low- and middle-income countries (LMICs), fewer than 5 percent of clinical trials are conducted in these regions.

This inequity not only limits access to potentially lifesaving treatments for local populations but also narrows the scope of research, often resulting in data that is less representative of global genetic and environmental diversity.

Expanding trials to LMICs has immense potential but is not without challenges. Countries must offer a stable rule of law, safety, and security to create a reliable environment for trial execution. Moreover, clinical sites need the infrastructure to meet the rigorous standards of clinical trials, including access to basic medical equipment, trained staff, and reliable systems for data collection and monitoring. Without these foundational elements, the quality and integrity of clinical trials can be compromised.

Despite these barriers, there are compelling examples of successful collaborations between high-income countries and LMICs that showcase the feasibility and benefits of conducting trials in diverse settings.

🔍 The Banner Alzheimer's Institute in Phoenix, Arizona, partnered with Colombian researchers to investigate a genetic form of early-onset Alzheimer's disease (EOAD) in families from Medellín, Colombia. This region is home to one of the largest populations with the Presenilin 1 (PSEN1) mutation, a genetic anomaly that virtually guarantees the development of Alzheimer's at an early age. The study enrolled participants who were mutation carriers but asymptomatic, testing the efficacy of an experimental drug aimed at preventing cognitive decline. This trial brought cutting-edge clinical trial opportunities to patients in Colombia but also exemplified how international collaboration can spearhead clinical innovation in LMICs. The study has generated invaluable insights into genetic Alzheimer's and highlighted the importance of conducting trials in regions where specific diseases are disproportionately represented.

Because certain conditions are highly prevalent in LMICs, these geographies present unique opportunities for research in both rare and frequent diseases. For instance, spinocerebellar ataxia type 2 (SCA2) is particularly common in Cuba due to a specific mutation that is significantly more frequent in this island; pantothenate kinase-associated neurodegeneration (PKAN, formerly known as Hallervorden-Spatz disease) has an unusually high prevalence in the Dominican Republic. Infectious diseases like malaria, dengue fever, and tuberculosis are endemic to many LMICs, providing opportunities to test vaccines and treatments in high-burden regions. Neglected tropical diseases such as Chagas, leishmaniasis, and schistosomiasis disproportionately affect LMICs yet receive minimal attention in high-income settings.

By addressing these challenges, researchers can ensure that clinical trials are representative, equitable, and scientifically rigorous.

Increased collaborations between high-income countries and LMICs can bring advanced medical innovations to underserved populations while enriching global healthcare with data that better reflects the diversity of humanity.

Decentralized Clinical Trials: Clinical Trials at (or Near) Home

The concept of decentralized clinical trials is reshaping how studies are conducted by shifting participation from research facilities to the patients' homes or their communities (e.g., their local pharmacy). This innovative model offers the potential to make trials more inclusive, convenient, and cost effective while maintaining the rigor required for regulatory approval.

What Are Decentralized Clinical Trials?

In traditional trials, participants travel to designated research sites for every test, drug administration, or monitoring visit. In decentralized trials, some of these activities are conducted remotely or locally, leveraging telemedicine, wearable devices, and home healthcare providers. Participants might receive study drugs by mail, complete digital diaries via smartphone apps, or have lab samples collected at home or at a nearby pharmacy. This minimizes logistical hurdles and allows individuals from remote or underserved areas to participate. Decentralized trials address several barriers that have historically hindered participation:

- Accessibility: Rural residents, those with mobility issues, and people with demanding schedules can now enroll without needing to travel extensively.

- Inclusivity: By broadening geographic reach, decentralized trials can improve representation, helping trials better reflect the real-world patient population.
- Retention: Reduced participant burden often translates to higher retention rates, ensuring more complete and robust data.
- Efficiency: Remote data collection and digital tools streamline operations, reducing the time and cost associated with running trials.

While the benefits are promising, decentralized trials face unique challenges. Data security and patient privacy are paramount as digital tools collect vast amounts of sensitive information. Ensuring that remote devices are accurate and reliable is another critical concern, as technological inconsistencies could skew results. Additionally, the regulatory framework for decentralized trials is still evolving. Questions about how to monitor adherence, ensure protocol compliance, and conduct virtual audits are ongoing. Sponsors and regulators must work together to create guidelines that uphold trial integrity without stifling innovation.

🔍 The ADAPTABLE trial, short for "Aspirin Dosing: A Patient-centric Trial Assessing Benefits and Long-term Effectiveness," stands out as a groundbreaking example of a decentralized trial. Its goal was to identify the optimal aspirin dose (81 mg vs. 325 mg) for preventing cardiovascular events in patients with a history of heart disease. What made this trial extraordinary was its fully decentralized design, one of the first of its kind at such a scale. Almost 500,000 individuals were approached online, of which 15,076 provided their consent electronically and were randomized remotely. The trial utilized a patient-centered research network and relied heavily on electronic health records (EHRs) for data collection, cutting costs significantly compared to traditional trials. Patients reported outcomes directly from their homes via a user-friendly digital interface, enabling real-time data submission without requiring clinic visits. This innovative model facilitated the participation of a diverse population across the United States while demonstrating the feasibility of reducing logistical barriers. The ADAPTABLE trial also showed how decentralized methods could make large-scale studies more efficient and cost effective, all while maintaining scientific rigor.

Similarly, during the COVID-19 pandemic, decentralized approaches enabled critical research to continue amid lockdowns. Trials for vaccines and treatments incorporated telemedicine visits and at-home testing kits, proving the model's adaptability.

The Path Forward

Decentralized trials are not a one-size-fits-all solution. Certain studies, such as those requiring complex imaging or invasive procedures (e.g., organ biopsies, colonoscopy), will still require in-person visits to the clinical trial sites or hospitals. However, hybrid trials, combining remote and site-based elements, are emerging as a flexible alternative.

As the infrastructure for decentralized trials improves, supported by advancements in wearables, AI, and secure data-sharing platforms, the clinical trial landscape will continue to evolve. This patient-centered model has the potential to democratize research, ensuring that lifesaving treatments are accessible to all.

AI and Digital Technologies

Although, in Chapter 3, we saw that currently available AI chatbots are not that useful to help find a clinical trial, a progressive integration of AI and digital technologies will likely revolutionize how clinical research is designed, conducted, and analyzed. The medical publications discussing cutting-edge applications of AI in clinical medicine are rapidly increasing.

AI is changing all drug development stages, not just clinical trials, by analyzing complex datasets such as genomics and proteomics to identify promising drug targets. For instance, AI can predict how a drug interacts with biological systems and streamline the process of identifying viable compounds. This approach has the potential to drastically reduce the time and cost required for early-stage drug discovery. However, even with these advancements, validation through traditional research methods remains critical to ensure safety and efficacy.

Specifically for clinical trials, AI and digital tools have the potential to reshape the landscape of clinical research, from recruitment to monitoring and data analysis. Let's explore how.

Using AI for Smarter Recruitment

AI algorithms can process large datasets and could be potentially used to identify eligible participants more effectively. By mining electronic health records (EHRs), social media activity, and genetic databases, AI could pinpoint potential participants who meet the specific criteria of a trial. For example, algorithms can be programmed to flag patients with rare genetic mutations or unusual disease presentations, expanding the reach of trials to include underrepresented populations.

🔍 In an open-label clinical trial evaluating two strategies to optimize heart failure treatment, researchers tested RECTIFIER (RAG-Enabled Clinical Trial Infrastructure for Inclusion Exclusion Review), an AI-powered system that combines Retrieval-Augmented Generation (RAG) with GPT-4, to improve recruitment. RECTIFIER assessed patients' clinical notes in electronic health records (EHRs) against thirteen specific inclusion and exclusion criteria. RECTIFIER achieved 98 percent accuracy in identifying eligible participants compared to 92 percent by human reviewers, demonstrating superior precision. Additionally, the AI system processed data significantly faster than humans, reducing both the time and costs associated with trial recruitment. This example underscores AI's transformative potential in clinical trial recruitment by improving accuracy, cost effectiveness, and scalability, particularly for large-scale studies.

Using AI for Trial Design Optimization

AI could potentially enhance the design phase of clinical trials by identifying novel, better endpoints, predicting results, and simulating millions of clinical trial scenarios. For example, machine learning models could analyze historical trial data to predict which variables are most likely to demonstrate a treatment's efficacy, allowing researchers to focus on those metrics. This could help streamline trials and reduce costs while maximizing their potential impact. Adaptive trial designs, enabled by AI, would allow researchers to modify protocols in real time based on interim results, leading to faster and more accurate conclusions.

Using AI for Improved Participant Monitoring

In addition to AI, technological advance is also impacting the development and use of digital tools or gizmos, such as wearable devices and smartphone apps. These can enable continuous monitoring of participants' health metrics, providing real-time data on vital signs, activity levels, and even medication adherence. These devices could enhance the accuracy of data collection in decentralized trials while reducing the burden on participants, who may no longer need to visit clinical sites as frequently. For example, a wearable device could monitor blood glucose levels or detect irregular heart rhythms, providing rich datasets that are far more comprehensive than sporadic in-clinic measurements.

Using AI for Improved Data Analysis of Endpoints

AI could analyze trial data in real time to improve the accuracy of the trial endpoints and assist human raters. This is particularly true in clinical trials in which the endpoint assessment requires specific skills, such as assessing images, for instance, of computerized tomography (e.g., reduction in the size of a tumor) or a histological sample from a biopsy.

🔍 Clinical trials for metabolic dysfunction-associated steatohepatitis (MASH), a liver condition linked to fat buildup and inflammation, often rely on microscopic examination of liver tissue obtained with a biopsy to decide who can join the study and to measure how well treatments work. This process depends on pathologists interpreting the biopsy samples, but human evaluations can vary significantly, which can affect trial outcomes. To address this challenge, researchers developed AIM-MASH, an AI tool designed to assist pathologists. AIM-MASH consistently aligned with expert opinions and proved as reliable as individual pathologists in assessing key liver damage markers. Its results were also highly consistent, reducing variability between human evaluations. Beyond matching human performance, AIM-MASH offered advantages like detecting subtle treatment effects in patients with advanced liver scarring, something that traditional methods often miss. For example, AIM-MASH revealed clearer differences in how well treatments reduced liver damage compared to placebo. This case highlights how AI can complement human expertise in clinical trials, improving consistency, reducing error rates, and providing more precise measurements of treatment success. Such innovations could help trials run more smoothly and yield more reliable results, ultimately benefiting patients by speeding up the development of effective therapies.

Using AI for Early Detection of Adverse Events

AI could monitor trial data in real time to improve the identification of potential safety concerns, ensuring quicker responses to potentially serious events. By analyzing diverse data streams, ranging from lab results to participant-reported symptoms, AI could identify early warning signs and mitigate risks more effectively than traditional monitoring systems.

🔍 An ST-elevation on an electrocardiogram (ECG) is an ominous marker indicating a heart attack (myocardial infarction), and early identification of such ST-elevations is critical to reducing mortality in affected patients. In an open-label, randomized controlled trial, researchers investigated the impact of AI-enabled ECG (AI-ECG) technology on reducing treatment delays for patients presenting with chest pain at a hospital in Taiwan. The trial enrolled 43,234 patients, evenly randomized into two groups: those assessed using AI-ECG technology and those receiving standard care. The AI-ECG system reduced the median time from hospital arrival to treatment of the heart attack by 14 minutes, lowering the time from 96 minutes in the control group to 82 minutes in the AI-ECG group. Importantly, the intervention group experienced fewer cases of cardiac death (85 versus 116). This study demonstrates the potential of AI in accelerating the identification of potentially fatal events. By reducing treatment delays, AI-ECG technology not only saves lives but also sets a precedent for integrating AI into both clinical trials and routine healthcare practices.

Ethical Considerations of AI in Clinical Trials

Like any powerful tool, AI comes with risks, some obvious, others lurking beneath the surface.

A major concern is privacy. AI-driven trials often require patient data to flow between hospitals, research institutions, and technology companies. While encryption and cybersecurity measures exist, every handoff increases the chance of data breaches, whether accidental or intentional. Patients may not always know where their information is going or how it's being used.

Then there's the issue of trust. AI isn't magic; it's an algorithm making predictions based on past data. But what happens if AI gets it wrong? Most AI models operate like a "black box," offering recommendations without clear explanations of how or why they came up with that recommendation. If a doctor relies too heavily on AI's suggestions or dismisses a patient's symptoms because they don't match the algorithm's predictions, mistakes could happen. Worse, over time, doctors could become too dependent on AI, losing critical diagnostic skills in the process.

Another ethical minefield is informed consent. Some AI-driven studies qualify for waivers of consent because they use preexisting medical data and, therefore, do not require new participants. This means your health records could be part of an AI trial without your knowledge. Even if a study poses minimal risk, the idea that your data could be used without your explicit permission raises serious ethical concerns. Shouldn't patients have the right to decide whether their health information is used to train an AI system?

Despite these challenges, it looks like AI is here to stay. The key is transparency: researchers must disclose when and how AI is involved, ensuring that both doctors and patients understand its strengths and limitations. With the right safeguards, AI could revolutionize clinical trials, not just by making them faster and cheaper but by making them smarter, fairer, and more centered on patients.

Could We Ever Get Rid of Clinical Trials?

While the idea of eliminating clinical trials is intriguing, it remains a distant, almost unimaginable possibility. Despite their limitations, the fact is that clinical trials remain essential for determining the safety and effectiveness of novel experimental therapies. However, these many limitations, such as high costs, long timelines, and ethical challenges (e.g., placebo), have spurred efforts to streamline or even bypass some aspects of the process.

So, could we at least minimize the role of clinical trials? The answer lies in a mix of innovations and constraints.

Advances in **real-world evidence (RWE)** are reshaping how treatments are evaluated. RWE involves analyzing data from everyday healthcare settings, such as electronic health records (EHRs), insurance claims, and patient registries, to assess how a drug performs in the real world. This approach can supplement clinical trials, offering insights into long-term safety and effectiveness across diverse populations. RWE is particularly useful in rare diseases and, as we have discussed previously, the FDA might sometimes allow using this type of data instead of placebo arms. However, RWE cannot yet fully replace the controlled environment of clinical trials, which are designed to isolate the effects of a specific intervention.

Another innovation is the increasing use of adaptive trial designs, as discussed before. These flexible designs can shorten trial durations and reduce the number of participants required, making the process more efficient.

AI-powered simulations, known as "in silico trials" or "virtual clinical trials," offer another avenue to reduce reliance on human trials. These models use virtual populations and computer simulations to predict drug behavior and interactions. Therefore, these models can simulate millions of different scenarios, including populations and trial designs. Regulatory agencies like the FDA have started accepting "in silico" data for some scenarios, but this approach is not yet advanced enough to replace human trials entirely.

Biomarkers, biological indicators such as imaging, blood tests, or genetic markers, can sometimes provide quicker insights into whether a treatment is working. For instance, in cancer clinical trials, tumor size reduction can often replace long-term outcomes, such as survival rates, and speed up trial timelines. However, reliance on biomarkers could be misleading if they do not fully capture the complexities of a disease.

Programs like the FDA's "Breakthrough Therapy Designation" and the European Medicines Agency's PRIME (Priority Medicines) initiative offer expedited review processes for promising therapies, often requiring fewer participants or shorter trials. These pathways, however, still demand rigorous evidence to ensure patient safety and efficacy.

Despite these advancements, there are significant reasons why traditional clinical trials in human participants remain indispensable:

- Human biology is complex, and unexpected side effects or interactions often emerge only during controlled testing in diverse populations.
- Introducing a drug to the public without thorough testing in clinical trials could lead to widespread harm, undermining public trust.

- Regulatory agencies like the FDA require robust data to ensure that treatments are safe and effective. Without clinical trials, meeting these standards would be nearly impossible.

So, while the complete elimination of clinical trials is unlikely, at least in the short and medium term, their role may evolve. Hybrid models that integrate real-world evidence, computational simulations, and decentralized designs could redefine how we evaluate treatments. The regulatory environment will also need to become more flexible and adapt, allowing innovations while ensuring patient safety—an arduous task.

For now, clinical trials remain the gold standard, but ongoing advancements aim to make them faster and cheaper, bringing us closer to a future where their burdens are significantly reduced.

The Most Important Innovation: Empowered Participants

Clinical trials have long been viewed as carefully controlled experiments: patients enroll, follow protocols, and await results. But today, that perception is changing. A quiet revolution is unfolding, one in which participants are no longer just data points in a study but active partners in discovery. And with that shift comes a fundamental truth: your voice matters.

The future of medicine is not written in laboratories alone. It is written in the courage of every person who chooses to participate in research, in the questions they ask, the experiences they share, and the advocacy they inspire. With each step forward, whether joining a trial, speaking out about the participant experience, or pushing for more patient-centered research, you are helping shape a new era of clinical science.

Staying informed is not just about making better decisions; it is about claiming ownership of your role in research. That means asking questions, demanding transparency, and understanding the ethical frameworks designed to protect you. It means knowing that informed consent is more than a form; it is a conversation, an ongoing dialogue where you always have the right to ask, challenge, and walk away.

And it also means recognizing that participation in a clinical trial, whether it leads to a breakthrough or not, is never in vain. Every person who takes part contributes to a greater body of knowledge that may save or improve lives in the future. Every moment spent in a study, every blood draw, every survey answered—it all matters.

No one should have to navigate clinical research alone. Organizations like CISCRP and other advocacy groups work to ensure that participants are heard and actively included in shaping the future of trials. Meanwhile, patient communities provide support, solidarity, and a reminder that your journey is part of something much larger than yourself.

Regulatory agencies like the FDA and EMA are also listening more closely than ever, ensuring that trials are not only scientifically rigorous but also ethically sound, patient friendly, and truly representative of the people they aim to help. The landscape is shifting, and the voices of participants are at the center of that transformation.

This book may be ending, but your journey does not. Whether you are a current participant, considering a trial, or simply advocating for more ethical and effective research, you are already part of something far greater than any single study.

Clinical research is not just about treatments or data; it is about hope. It is about people like you who choose to step forward, not just for themselves but for the millions who will come after them.

Your participation, your curiosity, and your advocacy shape the future of medicine. And when that future arrives, when someone receives a life-changing treatment because of the knowledge uncovered in trials like yours, you will have been part of that story.

That is a legacy worth leaving.

Chapter 9 Highlights

- The future of clinical trials is being shaped by innovation and patient empowerment, making research more efficient, accessible, and inclusive.

- Decentralized clinical trials reduce patient burden by enabling participation from home, leveraging telemedicine, wearable devices, and remote monitoring.

- AI is changing trial design, recruitment, and data analysis, although ethical concerns, such as data privacy, bias, and transparency, must be addressed.

- Smarter clinical trials, including those using real-world evidence and adaptive designs, aim to accelerate drug development without compromising scientific rigor.

- Patients are no longer just participants but partners in research, with advocacy organizations, digital tools, and regulatory shifts ensuring their voices shape the future of clinical trials.

Epilogue: Considering Clinical Trials—A Leap of Hope

I once struck up a conversation with an older gentleman during a layover at an airport cafeteria. When I shared what I did for a living, he told me about his work at a car repair business. Then, he said something that stuck with me: "You know, sometimes, when things go wrong at my shop, I get anxious. But then I think, 'Relax, you're not in a race to cure horrible diseases.'" He paused and added, "But here you are, in that very race!"

This gentleman captured it perfectly. Clinical trials are not just about complex, cutting-edge science. They are a serious, human endeavor at the heart of medical innovation. Thanks to these trials, we now have treatments that were once unimaginable, like pembrolizumab for cancer, imatinib for leukemia, and ibrutinib for lymphoma. Yet, it's vital to remember that behind every breakthrough is the courage and altruism of trial participants. Every treatment, drug, or device available today owes its existence to those who said "yes" to an uncertain path.

These volunteers, often motivated by hope or the desire to help others, have advanced science while facing significant risks. Vitally, clinical trial participants have also played a critical role in identifying unsafe or ineffective drugs before they reach the public. While much attention is given to treatments that succeed and later fail, it is less recognized how many potentially harmful drugs are halted in development thanks to early trial participants. Their experiences, some involving severe or even fatal side effects, save countless lives by preventing these drugs from entering the market. From the smallest first-in-human trials to the massive studies that redefine standards of care, clinical trial participants are truly the unsung heroes of modern medicine. Their contributions safeguard public health and shape the future of medical progress.

Participating in a clinical trial is not merely a personal decision; it is a profound leap of hope. Hope for oneself, for future patients, and for a better understanding of complex diseases. For those in desperate, life-threatening situations, a trial can represent a chance, however uncertain, to access cutting-edge therapies. For healthy volunteers, participation often stems from a selfless desire to contribute to science and society.

Behind the scenes, each participant becomes part of a vast and intricate process. They endure long hours, repeated tests, potential side effects, and the uncertainty of outcomes. Yet their contributions drive the knowledge that reshapes healthcare, bringing cures to previously untreatable diseases and relief to those in pain.

As discussed in previous chapters, it is essential to acknowledge that clinical trial participation is not without challenges. Participants navigate uncharted territory, facing emotional, physical, and logistical obstacles. The informed consent process, treatment protocols, and trial designs are rigorous by necessity. Yet, for every trial participant who perseveres, the ripple effects are immeasurable, touching the lives of countless others who may never know their names.

Looking ahead, the landscape of clinical trials is changing rapidly. Advances in AI, decentralized models, and innovative trial designs promise to reduce barriers and improve accessibility. Yet, these innovations must never overshadow the core human element. Participants are not just data points; they are individuals with families, aspirations, and dreams. Respect for their dignity and trust must remain paramount as we push the boundaries of medical science.

If you are considering joining a clinical trial, know that you are stepping into a legacy of courage and discovery. Whether or not the trial succeeds, your contribution helps lay the foundation for the medical breakthroughs of tomorrow. You are not just a subject in a study; you are a vital partner in the quest for better health for all.

Clinical trials are a testament to the resilience of the human spirit. They represent a collective leap of hope, a bridge between today's challenges and tomorrow's possibilities.

To all who have participated, or are considering participation, this book honors your bravery and commitment.

You are the heroes of medicine.

Acknowledgments

Writing this book has been a deeply rewarding endeavor, and I am grateful to the many individuals who contributed their time, insight, and support along the way.

I am especially thankful to my literary agent, Matt Wager, for believing in this project from the very beginning and for guiding it to publication. At Rowman & Littlefield (now Bloomsbury), I am indebted to Jacquie Flynn for her thoughtful editorial leadership, and to Mikayla Lindsay for her invaluable assistance throughout the process. Their care and commitment made this a better book.

I am also grateful to the many colleagues in academia, industry, and regulatory authorities, as well as to the patients and caregivers who have shared their experiences with clinical trials over the years. Their courage and candor have profoundly shaped my understanding of this complex and often challenging landscape. Without their willingness to share, participate, and teach, none of this work would be possible.

I would like to acknowledge Horacio Kaufmann, MD, Professor of Neurology, Medicine and Pediatrics, and Director of the Autonomic Disorders Division at the New York University Grossman School of Medicine. I had the privilege of training with him, and his mentorship encouraged me early on to develop a deep interest in clinical trial design, conduct, and ethics, especially in the context of devastating neurological disorders. His guidance shaped the trajectory of my career, leading to a faculty appointment at NYU, a later transition to the pharmaceutical industry, and ultimately, the writing of this book.

Finally, my deepest gratitude goes to my wife, whose patience, insight, and constant encouragement sustained me throughout the writing process, especially while managing our two young children so I could focus on typing these words.

Resources for Further Information

This curated list of trusted resources is designed to help you navigate the clinical trial landscape. It includes reliable information, trial search tools, and support networks for various conditions.

Understanding Clinical Trials

Beyond the information provided in this book, these resources provide information on how clinical trials work, patient rights, and ethical protections.

- Center for Information & Study on Clinical Research Participation (CISCRP)
  A nonprofit dedicated to educating and engaging patients about clinical trials.
  Website: www.ciscrp.org

- NIH Clinical Research Trials and You
  A patient-friendly guide explaining the clinical trial process, participant rights, and expectations.
  Website: www.nih.gov/health-information/nih-clinical-research-trials-you

- FDA Clinical Trials: What Patients Need to Know
  Covers trial regulations, patient protections, and the drug approval process.

Website: www.fda.gov/patients/clinical-trials-what-patients-need-know

Finding Clinical Trial

Use these resources to search for clinical trials based on location, condition, or treatment.

Major Trial Registries

- ClinicalTrials.gov
  The most comprehensive US and international clinical trial database.
  Website: www.clinicaltrials.gov

- EU Clinical Trials Register
  Covers trials conducted in the European Union.
  Website: www.clinicaltrialsregister.eu

- WHO International Clinical Trials Registry Platform (ICTRP)
  Aggregates global trial data from multiple national registries.
  Website: www.who.int/clinical-trials-registry-platform

Disease-Specific Trial Finders

- National Cancer Institute (NCI) Clinical Trials
  Specialized cancer trial search tool.
  Website: www.cancer.gov/about-cancer/treatment/clinical-trials

- National Institute of Mental Health (NIMH) Trials
  Mental health-specific clinical trial search tool.
  Website: www.nimh.nih.gov/health/clinical-trials

- Fox Trial Finder
  Parkinson's disease clinical trial-matching tool.
  Website: www.michaeljfox.org/fox-trial-finder

- Breast Cancer Trials
  Tailored trial searches for breast cancer patients.
  Website: www.breastcancertrials.org

- Cystic Fibrosis Foundation Clinical Trials Finder
  Cystic fibrosis-specific trial database.
  Website: www.cff.org/clinical-trials

Academic Medical Centers and Hospitals

Many leading research hospitals offer clinical trial search portals with local trial information and direct contact points.

- Memorial Sloan Kettering Cancer Center—Cancer trials
  Website: www.mskcc.org/cancer-care/clinical-trials

- MD Anderson Cancer Center—Cancer trials
  Website: www.mdanderson.org/patients-family/diagnosis-treatment/clinical-trials.html

- Mayo Clinic Clinical Trials—Multidisciplinary trials
  Website: www.mayo.edu/research/clinical-trials

- NYU Langone Health—Various medical specialties
  Website: www.clinicaltrials.med.nyu.edu

- Bascom Palmer Eye Institute—Ophthalmology trials
  Website: www.umiamihealth.org/en/bascom-palmer-eye-institute/research/clinical-trials

If you're already a patient at an academic medical center, check their website for condition-specific trials.

Pharmaceutical Company Trial Portals

Pharmaceutical companies often list ongoing clinical trials for their investigational drugs.

- Pfizer
  Website: www.pfizerclinicaltrials.com

- Novartis
  Website: www.novartisclinicaltrials.com

- Roche
  Website: www.roche.com/research_and_development/who_we_are_how_we_work/clinical_trials.htm

- Johnson & Johnson (Janssen)
  Website: www.janssen.com/clinical-trials

Advocacy and Support Organizations

These organizations provide patient support, trial navigation, and advocacy:

General Patient Advocacy

- Patient Advocate Foundation—Assists with trial logistics, financial concerns, and insurance issues.
  Website: www.patientadvocate.org

- National Organization for Rare Disorders (NORD)—Offers guidance and advocacy for rare disease patients.
  Website: www.rarediseases.org

- Global Genes—Education and networking for rare disease patients and families.
  Website: www.globalgenes.org

Cancer Support

- American Cancer Society (ACS)—Trial support and general cancer resources.
  Website: www.cancer.org
- Susan G. Komen Foundation—Breast cancer advocacy and trial navigation.
  Website: www.komen.org
- Leukemia & Lymphoma Society—Provides support for blood cancer patients and funds research.
  Website: www.lls.org

Cardiovascular Health

- American Heart Association (AHA)—Heart disease education and trial guidance.
  Website: www.heart.org
- WomenHeart—Heart health advocacy for women.
  Website: www.womenheart.org

Diabetes

- American Diabetes Association (ADA)—Diabetes education and trial information.
  Website: www.diabetes.org
- Juvenile Diabetes Research Foundation (JDRF)—Type 1 diabetes research and advocacy.
  Website: www.jdrf.org

Neurological Diseases

- Alzheimer's Association—Support and research updates for Alzheimer's patients and caregivers.
  Website: www.alz.org

- Michael J. Fox Foundation for Parkinson's Research—Parkinson's research and trial matching.
  Website: www.michaeljfox.org

- Epilepsy Foundation—Epilepsy patient support and advocacy.
  Website: www.epilepsy.com

- National Multiple Sclerosis Society—MS education and clinical trial support.
  Website: www.nationalmssociety.org

Lung Diseases

- American Lung Association—Support for lung disease patients and trial navigation.
  Website: www.lung.org

- COPD Foundation—Advocates for individuals with chronic obstructive pulmonary disease and related conditions.
  Website: www.copdfoundation.org

- Cystic Fibrosis Foundation—Advocacy and research funding for cystic fibrosis.
  Website: www.cff.org

Liver Diseases

- American Liver Foundation—Support for patients with liver diseases.
  Website: https://liverfoundation.org

Chronic Pain

- American Chronic Pain Association—Offers support and resources for individuals living with chronic pain.
  Website: www.theacpa.org

Autoimmune Disorders

- Arthritis Foundation—Advocates for individuals with arthritis and related conditions.
  Website: www.arthritis.org

- Lupus Foundation of America—Provides support and resources for lupus patients.
  Website: www.lupus.org

Digestive Disorders

- Crohn's & Colitis Foundation—Supports individuals with inflammatory bowel diseases.
  Website: www.crohnscolitisfoundation.org

- Celiac Disease Foundation—Advocates for individuals with celiac disease and gluten-related disorders.
  Website: www.celiac.org

Kidney Disorders

- National Kidney Foundation—Provides education and support for kidney health and disease prevention.
  Website: www.kidney.org

Skin Disorders

- National Psoriasis Foundation—Advocates for individuals with psoriasis and psoriatic arthritis.
  Website: www.psoriasis.org

Respiratory Disorders

- American Lung Association—Provides resources for lung health and disease prevention.
  Website: www.lung.org

- COPD Foundation—Advocates for individuals with chronic obstructive pulmonary disease.
  Website: www.copdfoundation.org

Special Populations: Women, Children, and Families

- NIH Office of Research on Women's Health (ORWH)—Ensures women's representation in clinical research.
  Website: www.orwh.od.nih.gov

- MotherToBaby—Provides evidence-based data on medication safety during pregnancy.
  Website: www.mothertobaby.org

- Children's Hospital of Philadelphia (CHOP)—Pediatric clinical trials guidance.
  Website: www.chop.edu/clinical-trials

- Ronald McDonald House Charities (RMHC)—Housing assistance for families of children receiving treatment.
  Website: www.rmhc.org

Transparency and Clinical Trial Results

- FDA Drug Approvals & Safety Information—Track newly approved drugs and safety updates.
  Website: www.fda.gov/drugs/drug-approvals-and-databases

- AllTrials Campaign—Advocacy for full disclosure of clinical trial data, ensuring both positive and negative results are reported.
  Website: www.alltrials.net

💡 Pro Tip: Many patient advocacy groups and academic hospitals have trial search tools specific to your condition. If you're considering participating, check multiple sources for the most up-to-date information.

Glossary

This glossary is designed to make the terminology used in this book clear and accessible. It includes key terms related to clinical trials, drug development, and regulatory processes, providing readers with concise, easy-to-understand definitions. While this glossary covers the most relevant terms discussed in the book, it may not include every specialized term you might encounter in clinical trial documents or discussions with investigators. If you come across an unfamiliar term in a trial-related document or conversation, don't hesitate to ask for clarification. Understanding the details is crucial when navigating clinical research.

***

adherence (also known as *compliance*): The extent to which participants follow study instructions, such as taking medications as directed. Poor adherence can impact study outcomes.

adverse effect: Harmful and undesirable outcomes that are directly caused by the drug. They can range from mild (like nausea) to severe (organ failure). Sometimes referred to as adverse drug reactions.

adverse event (AE): An unwanted or harmful effect experienced during a clinical trial, which may or may not be caused by the treatment being tested.

assent: In clinical research, assent refers to the affirmative agreement of a minor or cognitively impaired individual to participate in a study. Unlike consent (which is legally binding), assent recognizes that the individual understands the study to the best of their ability and agrees to take part. Parental or guardian consent is still required.

baseline: Initial health status of a participant before receiving the investigational treatment, used as a reference point for measuring treatment effects.

bias: A systematic error in study design or conduct that can affect results and conclusions.

biologics: A drug derived from living organisms, such as vaccines, monoclonal antibodies, or gene therapies.

biomarker: A measurable indicator of a biological condition or disease. It can be a substance, molecule, gene, or other measurable entity used to assess a disease state or response to treatment. Biomarkers are often used in clinical trials to evaluate the effectiveness of interventions or to predict disease progression. For example, elevated levels of cholesterol in the blood can serve as a biomarker for cardiovascular disease.

biotechnology: The use of biological systems or organisms to develop medical treatments and technologies.

blinding (also known as *masking*): A study design in which participants and/or researchers do not know who is receiving the active treatment or placebo.

clinical research: The study of health and disease in humans to develop new treatments, interventions, or medical knowledge.

clinical trial: A research study that evaluates the effect of an intervention (such as a drug, device, or procedure) on health-related outcomes in humans.

control group: A group of participants in a clinical trial that receives a placebo or standard treatment instead of the experimental treatment, allowing for comparison.

crossover design: A study design in which participants receive multiple treatments in a specific sequence, allowing each participant to serve as their own control.

Data Safety Monitoring Board (DSMB): An independent group of experts (clinicians, statisticians, sometimes ethicists) that monitors ongoing large or complex clinical trials for safety concerns, efficacy signals, and scientific integrity. The DSMB can recommend modifying, continuing, or stopping a trial based on interim data.

decentralized clinical trial: A clinical trial that incorporates remote or virtual elements, such as telemedicine visits, home monitoring, or local healthcare providers, reducing the need for in-person visits.

delayed-start design: A study design used to assess whether a treatment has a disease-modifying effect by comparing early and delayed treatment groups.

device (medical device): A medical instrument, machine, or implant used for diagnosis, treatment, or prevention of disease.

dissent: The explicit refusal of a minor or cognitively impaired individual to participate in a clinical trial. Even if a legal guardian provides consent, a child's or dependent adult's dissent should be respected unless there is an overriding medical justification.

double-blind study: A study design in which neither participants nor researchers know who is receiving the active treatment or placebo, preventing bias.

drug: A substance used to diagnose, treat, or prevent disease.

efficacy: The ability of a treatment to produce the desired effect under controlled conditions.

eligibility criteria: The specific requirements that determine whether a person can participate in a clinical trial.

endpoint: A key measurement in a clinical trial that determines whether a treatment is effective (e.g., survival rate, symptom improvement).

European Medicines Agency (EMA): The European agency responsible for regulating drugs, medical devices, and other health-related products.

exclusion criteria: Factors that disqualify a person from participating in a clinical trial.

Expanded Access Program (also known as *Compassionate Use*): A pathway allowing patients with serious conditions to access experimental treatments outside of a clinical trial.

Food and Drug Administration (FDA): The US agency responsible for regulating drugs, medical devices, and other health-related products.

formulation: The composition of a drug, including active and inactive ingredients, which affects how the drug is delivered and absorbed.

futility: A determination made during an interim analysis indicating that a trial is unlikely to achieve its intended goals, often leading to early termination of the study.

generic drug: A medication that has the same active ingredients, dosage, and effectiveness as a brand-name drug but is typically less expensive.

HIPAA (Health Insurance Portability and Accountability Act): A US law that protects patient health information and ensures individuals have the right to access their own medical records.

inclusion criteria: Factors that determine eligibility for participation in a clinical trial.

informed consent process: The process by which participants learn about the details, risks, and benefits of a clinical trial before deciding to enroll.

informed consent form (ICF): A document that explains a clinical trial's purpose, risks, and procedures, which participants must sign before enrolling.

institutional review board (IRB): An ethics committee that reviews and approves clinical trials to ensure participant safety and rights.

intervention: Any action taken in a clinical trial, such as administering a drug or changing a lifestyle factor, to assess its effects on health.

interventional trials: A type of clinical study in which participants receive an intervention, such as a new drug or procedure.

Investigational New Drug (IND) application: A request submitted to the FDA to begin human testing of a new drug.

investigator: A researcher or physician responsible for conducting a clinical trial at a study site. The physician or researcher overseeing the trial is the principal investigator (PI).

Medicare: A US government health insurance program primarily for people aged sixty-five and older.

new drug application (NDA): A request submitted to the FDA for approval to market a new drug.

nocebo effect: When negative expectations cause a participant to experience adverse effects unrelated to the actual treatment.

observational (noninterventional) study: A study in which researchers monitor participants without providing any specific intervention.

off-label prescribing: The prescription of a drug for a condition or population not specifically approved by regulatory agencies.

open-label extension: A study phase where all participants receive the active treatment after completing a blinded clinical trial.

outcome: The result or effect measured in a clinical trial to determine the treatment's impact.

orphan disease (*rare disease*)**:** A condition affecting a small population, often defined as fewer than 200,000 people in the United States.

orphan drug: A drug developed to treat a rare disease, often receiving regulatory incentives to encourage development.

pharmacokinetics (PK): The branch of pharmacology concerned with the movement of drugs within the body. It describes how the body absorbs, distributes, metabolizes, and excretes a drug. The core components of pharmacokinetics are commonly referred to as ADME: absorption (how the drug enters the bloodstream), distribution (how the drug is spread throughout the body's tissues and organs), metabolism (how the drug is broken down by the liver or other organs), and excretion (how the drug or its metabolites are eliminated, usually via urine or feces). Pharmacokinetics helps to determine the optimal dosing, timing, and formulation of an experimental drug.

placebo: A substance that is designed to look like the experimental treatment but has no therapeutic effect.

preclinical: The stage of drug development that occurs before human trials, involving laboratory and animal studies to assess safety and efficacy. In some contexts, it can also mean the stage of disease when the patient has not yet experienced clinical manifestations of the disease, as a synonym for presymptomatic.

principal investigator (PI): The lead researcher responsible for conducting and overseeing a clinical trial at a specific site.

protocol: The detailed plan outlining how a clinical trial is conducted, including objectives, design, and procedures.

protocol deviation: A departure from the approved study protocol, which may affect data integrity or participant safety. Significant, serious, or intentional deviations are referred to as protocol violations.

randomization: A process that assigns participants to different treatment groups by chance to reduce bias.

rare disease (also referred to as *orphan disease*)**:** A condition affecting a small percentage of the population.

real-world evidence (RWE): data derived from real-world settings outside of the controlled environment of clinical trials. This includes information gathered from routine clinical practice, patient registries, electronic health records (EHRs), insurance claims data, and other sources. RWE helps to understand how treatments perform in diverse, broader populations, providing insights into the effectiveness, safety, and utilization of therapies under real-world conditions. It can complement clinical trial data by offering a more comprehensive view of a drug's performance in everyday use.

repurposing (drug repurposing): The use of an existing drug for a new therapeutic purpose, potentially accelerating development timelines.

research coordinator: A professional who manages day-to-day clinical trial operations, including participant communication and data collection.

risk-benefit ratio: An evaluation of the potential benefits of a treatment compared to its potential risks.

safety: The assessment of potential harm or adverse effects associated with an intervention.

screen failure: When a participant does not meet eligibility criteria during the screening process and cannot enroll in the trial.

screening: The initial phase of a clinical trial in which participants are evaluated for eligibility.

serious adverse event (SAE): A significant medical event that results in hospitalization, disability, or death.

sham procedure: A fake or inactive intervention used to create a control group in studies evaluating non-drug (typically surgical) treatments.

sponsor: The organization responsible for funding and overseeing a clinical trial.

standard of care: The best available treatment currently accepted by the medical community.

therapeutic target: The specific structure of the body (or, in the case of antibiotic therapies, the illness-causing germ) that a medicine is designed to interact with, with the goal of ameliorating symptoms or slowing/stopping the disease. This includes, for instance, a key protein or enzyme, a cell surface receptor, or a genetic mutation in your DNA.

tolerability: The degree to which participants can handle the side effects of a treatment.

unblinding: The process by which participants or researchers in a clinical trial become aware of which treatment group (e.g., placebo or active drug) the participant is assigned to. Intentional unblinding typically happens at the end of the trial or in emergencies, and it must be done carefully to maintain the integrity of the data. Unintentional unblinding can occur if the trial is poorly designed or when participants or researchers deviate from the protocol.

Selected Bibliography

Key Guidelines, Policy Documents

Food and Drug Administration. *E6(R2) Good Clinical Practice: Integrated Addendum to ICH E6(R1)*. Washington, DC: U.S. Food and Drug Administration, March 1, 2018.
National Commission for the Protection of Human Subjects of Biomedical and Behavioral Research. *The Belmont Report: Ethical Principles and Guidelines for the Protection of Human Subjects of Research*. Washington, DC: U.S. Government Printing Office, 1979. https://www.hhs.gov/ohrp/regulations-and-policy/belmont-report/index.html.
World Medical Association. "Declaration of Helsinki: Ethical Principles for Medical Research Involving Human Subjects." *Journal of the American Medical Association* 310, no. 20 (2013): 2191–94.

Seminal Publications on Clinical Trials

Emanuel, Ezekiel J., Christine C. Grady, Robert A. Crouch, Reidar K. Lie, Franklin G. Miller, and David Wendler, eds. *The Oxford Textbook of Clinical Research Ethics*. 1st ed. New York: Oxford University Press, 2008.
Emanuel, Ezekiel J., Robert A. Crouch, et al., eds. *Ethical and Regulatory Aspects of Clinical Research: Readings and Commentary*. 1st ed. Baltimore: Johns Hopkins University Press, 2004.
Friedman, Lawrence M., Curt D. Furberg, and David L. DeMets. *Fundamentals of Clinical Trials*. 4th ed. New York: Springer, 2010.
Zarin, Deborah A., Tony Tse, Rebecca J. Williams, and Nicholas J. Califf. "Clinical Trial Registration and Results Reporting: Evolution of Legal and Ethical Requirements." *New England Journal of Medicine* 375, no. 20 (2016): 1998–2004. https://doi.org/10.1056/NEJMra1510055.

Historical Sources

Alexander, Leo. "Medical Science under Dictatorship." *New England Journal of Medicine* 241, no. 2 (1949): 39–47. https://doi.org/10.1056/NEJM194907142410201.

Beecher, Henry K. "Ethics and Clinical Research." *New England Journal of Medicine* 274, no. 24 (1966): 1354–60.

Washington, Harriet A. *Medical Apartheid: The Dark History of Medical Experimentation on Black Americans from Colonial Times to the Present*. New York: Doubleday, 2006.

Patient Participation and Empowerment

Appelbaum, Paul S., Charles W. Lidz, and Robert Klitzman. "Voluntariness of Consent to Research: A Preliminary Empirical Investigation." *IRB: Ethics & Human Research* 31, no. 6 (November–December 2009).

Berg, J. W., Paul S. Appelbaum, Charles W. Lidz, and Lisa Parker. *Informed Consent: Legal Theory and Clinical Practice*. 2nd ed. New York: Oxford University Press, 2001.

Brody, David S. "The Patient's Role in Clinical Decision-Making." *Annals of Internal Medicine* 93, no. 5 (November 1980): 718–22. https://doi.org/10.7326/0003-4819-93-5-718.

Sacristán, José A., Antonio Aguarón, Carlos Avendaño-Solá, Pilar Garrido, Javier Carrión, Ana Gutiérrez, Roos Kroes, and Ainhoa Flores. "Patient Involvement in Clinical Research: Why, When, and How." *Patient Preference and Adherence* 10 (April 2016): 631–40. https://doi.org/10.2147/PPA.S104259.

Technology and the Future of Trials

Topol, Eric J. *The Creative Destruction of Medicine: How the Digital Revolution Will Create Better Health Care*. New York: Basic Books, 2012.

Underhill, Craig, et al. "Decentralized Clinical Trials as a New Paradigm of Trial Delivery to Improve Equity of Access." *JAMA Oncology* 10, no. 4 (2024): 526–30.

Yang, Anna H., and Isaac R. Rodriguez-Chavez, eds. *Fundamentals of Decentralized Clinical Trials: Strategy and Execution*. 1st ed. New York: Springer, 2024.

Index

adaptive trial design 224, 233–234, 241, 245
adherence 2, 15, 150, 210, 218, 241; see also noncompliance
adrenoleukodystrophy (ALD) 116
adverse events 14, 22, 28, 46, 159, 177, 243; see also safety; tolerability; risk-ratio.
advocacy groups see patient advocacy groups
Alzheimer's disease 34, 44, 47, 71, 102, 138, 141, 145, 165, 201, 236
amyotrophic lateral sclerosis (ALS) 67, 68, 113
antisense oligonucleotide 93–94
appreciation of trial participants 192–193
approval see drug approval process
Artificial Intelligence (AI)
   as tool for finding trials 77–79
   as tool for obtaining information on experimental therapies 106–108
   as tool for obtaining information on diseases 115–116
   ethical considerations 244–245
   in trials 231, 239–245
     for data analysis 242–243
     for participant monitoring 241–242
     for recruitment 240–241
     for trial design 241
     for safety surveillance 243
   Asian populations 227–228
assent 211

Barbershop Study 226
baseline visit 144–146; see also randomization
bespoke therapies 92
bias 53–54
biomarkers 14, 54
blinding 50, 53–54, 151; see also unblinding
burden of participation 46, 48–50, 92, 158, 166, 174, 198; see also financial burden and planning; travel considerations; scheduling; emotional aspects of participation

cancer 2, 15, 29, 48, 53, 66, 69, 104, 110, 113–114, 172, 209, 251
   relevance of disease stage 68
   relevance of genetic mutations 68, 114
   relevance of histological type 67
   search tools for breast cancer 82–83

caregivers
  as advocates 170
  emotional support by 170
  logistical support by 169
  support for 171–172
case studies (real-life)
  Emily Whitehead (CAR-T therapy) 38–39
  Jesse Gelsinger (OTC gene therapy) 39–40
  Josh Hardy (adenoviral infection) 40–41
  Terry Horgan (DMD gene therapy) 40
Center for Information and Study on Clinical Research Participation (CISCRP) 43, 48, 192, 195, 199, 248
ChatGPT see AI (artificial intelligence)
clinical development see clinical trial
clinical research 7, 130
clinical trial
  catastrophic accidents in trials 22, 252
  definition 8–14
  duration 110
  delays and cancellations 122–126
  funding 101, 124–125
  oversight 29–32
  participation 2, 42, 65
    barriers to participation 1–2
    benefits of participation 43–45
    risks of participation 46–50, 101
  phases 16–22, 104
    phase 1 (first-in-human) 17–18
    phase 2 18–19
    phase 3 19–20
    other phases (phase 0, phase 4) 20–21

ClinicalTrials.gov
  interpreting listings 70–77
  overview 70–71
  search functions 71–72
  study overview and summary 74
communication
  with clinical trial team 117, 148, 152, 203
  with primary physician 58–62
compliance see adherence
condition see indication
consent see informed consent
control
  control group 43
  control intervention 12
COVID-19 pandemic 22–23, 44, 121
criteria (inclusion and exclusion) see eligibility

data access see results
Data Safety Monitoring Board (DSMB) see safety, DSMB oversight
decentralized clinical trials 34, 237–239, 241
devices, regulatory approval 12
discontinuing a trial see withdrawal from a trial
diversity see representation
double blind see blinding
double dipping see fraud and scams
drug approval process 26–28, 185, 191, 223–224, 228
drug development process cost 25
drug discovery 25
drug repurposing
  definition 24
  examples (Viagra, aspirin, finasteride) 24–25

eligibility 100–101, 119–121,
    139, 141–143; see
    also informed consent;
    vulnerable populations;
    randomization
emotional aspects of participation
    49–50
empowerment 45, 247–249 see
    also participation; patient
    advocacy groups; informed
    consent.
end-of-study visit 181–184
endpoints 54
ethics committees see IRB
European Medicines Agency
    (EMA) 29
exclusion criteria see eligibility
expanded access program (EAP)
    88–90, 191
experimental therapy 113–116

financial burden and planning 49,
    158–163
    financial assistance 160–161
    impact on participation
        48–49, 163
    out-of-pocket costs 91, 159, 160
    tax deductions 161–162
first-in-human trial see clinical trial,
    phases, phase 1
Food and Drug Administration (FDA)
    9, 26–27, 29, 123, 130, 177
fraud and scams 94–97
    double dipping 29

gene therapy 23, 39, 53, 113
grapefruit 133

health goals 100, 121
Health Insurance Portability
    and Accountability Act
    (HIPAA) 120

health-related outcomes 13–14
healthy volunteers 13, 17–18, 22, 33,
    95, 252

important questions to ask yourself
    57–58
inclusion and exclusion criteria see
    eligibility
indication 103
informed consent 96, 130–134
    exceptions 138–139
informed consent form 118, 131
    content 135–136
    signature 136
    understanding 134
informed consent process 130
Institutional Review Board (IRB)
    30–31, 137
insurance see financial burden and
    planning
intervention 10–12
    control intervention see control
    interventional trial 71
    non-pharmacological
        intervention 10
    psychological intervention 13
intolerance see tolerability

location 70, 72, 75, 79, 82, 109
logistics see scheduling and travel
    considerations
Lorenzo's oil 116
low- and middle-income countries
    (LMICs) 235–237

medical devices see devices
medical history and medical
    records 139
Medicare 9
mental health disorders see
    vulnerable populations
missing a trial visit 146, 150

monitoring 14, 17, 21, 27, 43–46, 90–91, 146, 150, 154, 169, 183, 216, 219, 241, 243 see also DSMB
motivation for participation see clinical trial, participation, benefits of participation
myths about clinical trials 32–34

NCT number 73, 103
National Cancer Institute (NCI) 82
negative trial results see results
noncompliance 147, 150
noninterventional (observational) study 7–8, 71
n-of-1 trials 224

objective (primary objective of a trial) 100; see also health-related outcomes
off-label prescription 209
open-label extension (OLE) 47–48, 184–189
　pros and cons of OLE participation 188–189
Orphan Drug Act 222–223
　orphan drug exclusivity 223
out-of-pocket costs see financial burden and planning
outcomes see health-related outcomes

Parkinson's disease 7, 68–69, 71–72, 74–75, 82, 115, 142, 159
　placebo effect in 51–52
participation in clinical trials, see clinical trials, participation; burden of participation; empowerment; withdrawal from a trial
patient advocacy groups 82–83, 176

patient empowerment see empowerment
pediatric populations see vulnerable populations, children
pharmacokinetics 18
phases of clinical trials see clinical trial, phases
physical examination 139
placebo 47, 50–52 see also sham procedure; blinding
　placebo effect 51–52
　unethical use 52–53
post-market surveillance 28
preclinical studies (animal studies) 13, 26, 232–233
preliminary data 105
prescreening 119–121
primary physician
　communication with 58–62
principal investigator (PI) 28, 118
　responsibilities 28
protocol 147
　amendment 123
　deviation 149, 152
public health emergency see COVID-19 pandemic

questionnaires in a trial 140–141, 146, 150

randomization 12, 54–56, 144–145
ranking strategy for trials 76, 103–111
rare diseases 12, 221–225
real-world data (RWD) 224, 245
regulatory agencies 20, 177, 216, 228; see also FDA; EMA
representation in trials 225–228
repurposing see drug repurposing
rescreening 143–144
resilience 204

results
  integration into healthcare 199–201
  negative results 197–198
  participant access to 193–198
Right-to-Try law 90–91
risk–benefit ratio 15–16

safety see also adverse events; risk–benefit ratio; tolerability
  Data Safety Monitoring Board (DSMB) oversight 31–32
  definition 14
  in device approval process 13
  monitoring and reporting of 14, 16–19, 21–22
  participant role in ensuring 151–152, 177
  post-marketing safety surveillance 27–28
  responsibility for safety (regulatory and investigator roles) 28–31
  risks to participant safety 46
  safety concerns resulting in trial termination 125
  safety in vulnerable and unique populations 208–218, 227–228.
scheduling of trial visits 48–49, 101, 121, 123, 135, 142, 145–146, 150, 152, 155, 164–166, 168–169 see also missing a trial visit; travel considerations; burden of participation
  coordination with caregivers or travel plans 168–169
  impact on participation burden 48–49, 164–166
  managing conflicts 150, 155

screening and eligibility 121–124, 129–130, 136, 139–144, 145, 151 see also eligibility; prescreening; rescreening
screening visit 121–124, 129–130, 136, 139–140, 142–143, 145, 151
screen failure 143–144
searching and selecting clinical trials see also ClinicalTrials.gov; trial-matching platforms
  registries 79–82
  patient advocacy groups 82–83
  hospitals and research centers 83–84
  pharmaceutical companies 84
  social media 85
  ranking and selection strategy 100, 103–111
sham procedure 52; simulated treatment used for control purposes; see also placebo
side effects see adverse events; safety
spinal muscular atrophy (SMA) 23–24
sponsor 28, 108–109
spreadsheet see ranking strategy for trials
stage of disease 67
standard of care 9, 12, 69, 158 see also control intervention
statins 25–26, 33
support networks 167–175 see also patient advocacy groups; empowerment; emotional aspects of participation
  family and caregivers 167–172
  online communities 174–175
  advocacy groups 176

telemedicine 121, 146, 164, 239; see also decentralized trials
termination or delay of trials 122–125
    administrative causes 123, 125
    participant impact 125–126
    safety concerns resulting in 125
thalidomide 215–216
therapeutic target 112–113
tolerability 14–15
    definition 14
    withdrawal due to intolerance 46, 153; see also withdrawal from a trial
travel considerations 48–49, 122, 159, 163–166
trial assessments 140, 145
trial-matching platforms 85–87
trial myths see myths about clinical trials
trial phases see clinical trial, phases

unblinding 52, 54
uncertainty in trials 57–58
unique populations see vulnerable populations

Viagra see drug repurposing, examples
violation (protocol) 177
Vioxx (rofecoxib) 27–28
vulnerable populations
    children 208–215
        ethical considerations in pediatric trials 210–212
        questions to ask before a pediatric trial 213–215
    pregnant women 215–217
    elderly 217–218
    mental-health disorders 219–220
    prisoners 220–221
    orphan diseases see rare diseases

withdrawal from a trial 153–155 see also tolerability; termination or delay of trials.

younger patients see vulnerable populations

Zolgensma (SMA gene therapy) 23, 24, 53, 113

About the Author

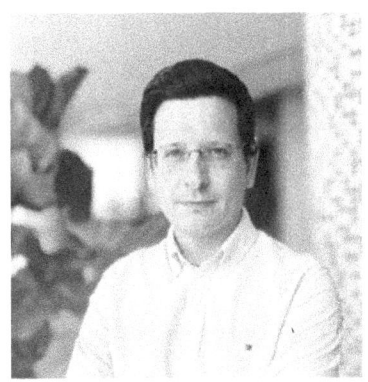

Dr. Jose-Alberto Palma. Credit: Pilar Gallardo

Dr. Jose-Alberto Palma, MD, PhD, FAAN, is a distinguished neurologist and neuroscientist with over a decade of groundbreaking experience in clinical trials and drug development. As an attending physician at New York University (NYU) Langone Health and Professor of Neurology at the NYU Grossman School of Medicine, Dr. Palma spearheaded transformative clinical trials for neurodegenerative disorders and authored more than two hundred peer-reviewed publications in leading biomedical journals. His extensive work with patients and caregivers has given him unique insight into the profound impact of clinical research. Dr. Palma later brought his expertise to developing medicines, assuming leadership roles at top pharmaceutical companies, first at Novartis and currently at Eli Lilly. In these roles, he has been at the forefront of designing global clinical trial strategies with innovative medicines for Alzheimer's, Parkinson's, and other neurodegenerative disorders. Alongside his work in the pharmaceutical industry, he has maintained a part-time faculty appointment at NYU, mentoring aspiring physicians and scientists and fostering collaborative research efforts. Dr. Palma's work, *A Patient's Guide for Clinical Trials*, reflects his passion for making clinical trials accessible and patient centered. He lives in Florida with his wife and two children.